Tissue Engineering Intelligence Unit 5

Biomaterials in the Design and Reliability of Medical Devices

Michael N. Helmus
Material Sciences Center
Boston Scientific Corporation
Natick, Massachusetts

Landes Bioscience / Eurekah.com
Georgetown, Texas
U.S.A

Kluwer Academic / Plenum Publishers
New York, New York
U.S.A

BIOMATERIALS IN THE DESIGN AND RELIABILITY OF MEDICAL DEVICES

Tissue Engineering Intelligence Unit 5

Landes Bioscience / Eurekah.com
and
Kluwer Academic / Plenum Publishers

Printed in the U.S.A.

Kluwer Academic / Plenum Publishers, 233 Spring Street, New York, New York, U.S.A. 10013
http://www.wkap.nl/

Please address all inquiries to Landes Bioscience / Eurekah.com:
Landes Bioscience / Eurekah.com, 810 South Church Street, Georgetown, Texas, U.S.A. 78626
Phone: 512/ 863 7762; FAX: 512/ 863 0081; www.Eurekah.com; www.landesbioscience.com
Landes tracking number: 1-58706-039-6

Biomaterials in the Design and Reliability of Medical Devices, edited by Michael N. Helmus, Landes / Kluwer dual imprint/ Landes series: Tissue Engineering Intelligence Unit 5,
ISBN 0-306-47690-8

Library of Congress Cataloging-in-Publication Data

CIP applied for but not received at time of publication.

Dedication

To my coauthors, coworkers, and colleagues and those special mentors in my career: Drs. Don Gibbons, Roger Snyder, and Mr. Josh Tolkoff. However, the most important are my family who have learned to live with my quirks and humor—my wife Shoshana, and daughters Devorah, Esther, and Rivkie. And in the memory of my parents who gave me the ability to pursue my dreams—Herbert and Bernice Helmus.

CONTENTS

Preface viii

1. **Overview and Introduction: Unique Aspects of Biomaterials in the Safety and Efficacy of Medical Implant Devices** 1
Michael N. Helmus
Materials Selection 1
Functional Requirements 2
Biomaterials and Regulatory Guidelines 53

2. **Standards and Guidelines for Biocompatibility of Medical Devices** 74
Sharon J. Northup
Product Registration Requirements 74
Standards and Guidelines for Biocompatibility Testing 106
Chemical Characterization 107
Risk Assessment 113
Case Studies of Materials Toxicity Risk Assessment 117
Conclusion 125

3. **Regulation of Medical Devices** 127
Barry Sall
U.S. Food and Drug Administration Regulation of Medical Devices 127

4. **Nonclinical Medical Device Testing** 144
Sharon J. Northup
Overview of Biocompatibility Procedures 144
Sample Preparation 146
Detailed Description of Biocompatibility Procedures 148
Cytotoxicity 149
Sensitization 150
Irritation Assays 152
Systemic Toxicity (Single and Repeated Dose Toxicity Including Pyrogenicity) 152
Pyrogenicity 156
Genotoxicity 157
Implantation 160
Hemocompatibility 162
Chronic Toxicity and Carcinogenicity 164
Reproductive and Developmental Toxicity 165
Biodegradation 165
Toxicokinetic Studies 166
Effectiveness Testing 167
Externally Communicating Devices 169
Implanted Devices 169
Conclusion 170

5. **Failure Analysis: Learning for the Future from the Past** 172
Michael N. Helmus

6. **Product Development in a Small Company Environment** 178
Roger W. Snyder
Records and Record Keeping 179
Testing 181
Materials and Components 182
Prototyping 184
Vendor Relationships 185
Sterilization and Shelf Life 186
Production Facilities 187
Conclusion 189

7. **Tissue Engineering Constructs and Commercialization** 191
Kelvin G.M. Brockbank
Case Studies: Development of Effective Transport Solutions and Devices to Enable Product Distribution 194
Development of Methods to Increase Product Shelf-life 195

8. **Testing of Biomaterials Modified with Bioactive Molecules: A Case Study** 198
Katherine S. Tweden
Characterization of the Nature and Uniformity of the Modification 199
Quantitation of the Modification 202
Assessment of the Biological Activity In Vitro 202
In Vitro Challenges 204
Manufacturing Ruggedness 204
Assessment of the Biological Activity In Vivo 205
Immobilization of an RGD-Containing Peptide: A Case Study 206
Materials 206
Results 209

Appendix: Selecting Contract Labs 223
Barry Sall

Index 224

EDITOR

Michael N. Helmus
Material Sciences Center
Boston Scientific Corporation
Natick, Massachusetts
Chapters 1, 5

CONTRIBUTORS

Kelvin Brockbank
Organ Recovery Systems
Charleston, South Carolina
Chapter 7

Sharon Northup
Northup Regulatory Toxicology Service
Highland Park, Illinois
Chapters 2, 4

Barry Sall
Worldwide Regulatory Affairs Services
PAREXEL International Corporation
Waltham, Massachusetts
Chapter 3, Appendix

Roger Snyder
Technical Services and Regulatory Affairs
LVAD Technology, Inc.
Detroit, Michigan
Chapter 6

Katherine Tweden
HeartStent Corporation
Brooklyn Park, Minnesota
Chapter 8

PREFACE

The implant was injection molded from a new elastic block copolymer. Water absorbed to the slightly hydrophilic backbone of the soft segment. Though the material passed all biocompatibility and safety tests, it did leach a slightly cytotoxic additive resulting in a mild chronic inflammatory response. White cells loomed and adhered to the surface. The cellular response over time resulted in the continual bathing of the material with low concentrations of lytic enzymes and a slightly acidic pH. The corner of the device was subject to a tensile bending stress. Below the surface of the implant, a craze, the beginnings of a microcrack had formed. The presence of water and the slightly acidic pH combined with the mild catalysis of the enzymes result in a slow but continuing degradation of the soft segments. As the implant experienced cyclic loading, microcracks coalesced. The onslaught of time continued, a crack formed. Joe was at work, his eyes opened wide....

Is this a Robin Cook nightmare in the making? The responsibility of medical device designers and engineers is to eliminate the sites of failure and to test the device and its materials of fabrication to demonstrate its ultimate safety and efficacy. The nightmare could occur if testing fails to account for synergistic interactions from chronic loading, aqueous environments, and biologic interactions. Testing methodologies are readily available to assess accelerated effects of loading in physiologic-like environments. This combined with the sub-chronic effects of animal implants is a potent tool in assessing durability. It is difficult to predict the chronic effects of the total biologic environment. The ultimate determination of safety comes not only from following the details of regulations, but with an understanding of potential failure modes and designs that lower risk of these failures. This is our challenge.

Biomaterials are an integral part of medical devices, implants, controlled drug delivery systems, and tissue engineered constructs. Extensive research efforts have been expended on understanding how biologic systems interact with biomaterials. Furthermore, efforts are now focused on how biologic interactions can be controlled by bioactive surfaces, nano-textures, nano-engineered surfaces, and hybrid systems containing cells. Meanwhile, controversy has revolved around biomaterials and their availability in traditional medical devices as a result of the backlash to huge liability resulting from such controversies as silicone gel escape from mammary prostheses and fragmentation of a temporomandibular joint implant fabricated from a composite of FEP (fluorinated ethylene polypropylene) and carbon fiber. Congress has passed the Biomaterials Availability Act to help address availability issues and the National Research Council has convened a Biomaterials Roundtable to address a wide range of technical and regulatory issues relating to improving biomaterials, testing, and availability for developing new medical devices and technology. This book specifically addresses the unique role of biomaterials in medical device design and the use of emerging biomaterials technology in medical devices. Unique challenges faced by small medical device businesses with respect to biomaterials, availability and testing are also addressed. Case studies in a small medical device environment are given. The case study given for bioactive materials is an excellent example of the challenges and innovativeness required in testing new materials. This book is a bridge between the academic and industrial worlds and provides guidelines and sources of information not readily tabulated in current texts.

Michael N. Helmus

CHAPTER 1

Overview and Introduction:
Unique Aspects of Biomaterials in the Safety and Efficacy of Medical Implant Devices

Michael N. Helmus

Biomaterials include a broad range of materials that must meet stringent and diverse requirements to be acceptable for use in the body and to meet the needs of specific devices. Biomaterials can be categorized as synthetic polymers (nonbiodegradable and biodegradable polymers); biologically derived materials (e.g., crosslinked xenografts); bioderived macromolecules; coatings (passive and bioactive); tissue adhesives; metal alloys; ceramics and carbons. Applications include blood-contacting devices and implants, soft tissue devices for repair and soft tissue reconstruction, orthopedic devices to aid bone repair and replace damaged bone and joints, and wound dressings for large area damage to skin from trauma, ulcers and burns. Evolving applications include the scaffolding for tissue regeneration and replacement as part of hybrid artificial organs and bioengineered tissues. Acceptable scaffolding materials for tissue engineered devices will need to not only be biocompatible in the traditional sense by allowing cellular interactions that result in tissue that mimics the naturally occurring material for which it will substitute but also from a biochemical and biomechanical perspective. Tissue engineered devices have a design requirement that the physical properties of the device meet the necessary requirements immediately and that they are maintained as either bioerodable scaffolds that are resorbed or that the tissue remodels. Tissue engineered devices may be formed on substrates of biodegradable polymers or on decellularized allografts or xenografts. Recellularization can be performed in a bioreactor or occur in situ. Growth factors and bioactive agents may be incorproated into the substrates to encourage the proper cell attachment and function. Furthermore, as living structures, adverse tissue responses such as hyperplastic responses need to be mitigated.

Materials Selection

The materials comprising the device, as fabricated and sterilized, must be nontoxic, noncarcinogenic, nonantigenic, and nonmutagenic. Devices for use in blood have a thromboresistance requirement, while there are noncardiovascular applications where the device may have a need to act as a hemostatic agent. The effect of a foreign body in vivo is essentially the study of wound healing in the presence of a sterile foreign material within the environment that it is placed, e.g., soft tissues, blood, neural tissue or bone. The outcome of this healing process can have profound implications on the success of a device and can be dependent on material properties. Its fatigue resistance and its biostability will determine the durability of the device. The biologic and physical criteria need to be evaluated in the context of the entire

Biomaterials in the Design and Reliability of Medical Devices, edited by Michael N. Helmus

device, its application, duration of use, and how it interfaces with the body. Basic schemes for testing the acceptability of materials in terms of cytotoxicity, hemolysis, and mutagenicity can be found in the following standards and guidelines: American Society for Testing and Materials (ASTM) F-748, the Tripartite Biocompatibility Guidance Document, and the International Standards Organization 10993-1 standard. The FDA implemented use of International Standard ISO-10993, "Biological Evaluation of Medial Devices—Part 1: Evaluation and Testing. However, the guideline is to be used with a FDA-modified matrix and Biocompatibility Flow Chart, Figure 3.1. These documents provide a method of testing by device application. ASTM Committee F04 is developing a standard for Tissue Engineered Medical Products that encompasses Normal Biological Function, Structural Characterization, Tissue Engineered Biomaterials, Biomolecules, Cells, Delivery Systems, Clinical Trials and Microbiological Safety.

The ability to select appropriate materials for a medical device involves a detailed knowledge of the requirements of the device, knowledge of materials, and predicate uses and failure modes, summarized in Tables 1.1, 1.2, 1.3. This provides the format for the basis of the book and how materials selection and analysis are related to the device and regulatory environment. Table 1.2 provides a guide to isolating the types of biomaterials related tests that are appropriate for a particular device and application within the context of device regulations.

Functional Requirements

Identification of a device's design intent and tissue interface will determine not only the regulatory requirements and safety tests, but also specific testing to demonstrate efficacy. FDA guidance documents provide detailed approaches for testing requirements of specific devices. Design intent will have a strong influence on the physical and biologic properties required as well as the test program required to demonstrate safety and efficacy. Specific constraints on the device and materials of construction may be imposed by the surgical and medical conditions of the patient. Table 1.3 summarizes these design considerations for implants. This also illustrates the range of polymeric and biologic materials utilized in medical devices: elastomers, gels, biologics, and drug release devices.

Nonimplantable devices such as blood contacting catheters demonstrate requirements in terms of soft tissue contact, blood contact, inflammation, infection, thrombosis, and intimal hyperplasia (i.e., thickening of the inner surface of the blood vessel). Design characteristics influence material selection decisions in order to meet characteristics of compliance (that is the opposite of stiffness), push, torque, and inflation of high pressure balloons. Many times the ability to meet different functional needs result in contradictory requirements and this may necessitate giving up one property in order to meet a high priority requirement.

Blood contacting catheters present an excellent example of functionality requirements of acute and semichronic (contact time of days to months) devices. The requirements for blood contact and soft tissue contact will be similar for both the semi-chronic and permanent implants. The differences are delineated on the FDA Blue Book use of ISO 10933 (see Chapter 3). The main differences in evaluation will be the length of time for biocompatibility implant testing. These devices have soft-tissue and blood contact requirements as well as safety and efficacy demands. Trade-offs can be seen in the need to limit intimal damage of the blood vessels by having a soft nature. However, the ability to place and rotate, i.e., torque, the catheter requires longitudinal and radial stiffness. The tortuous nature of blood vessels and the long length to reach treatment sites impose more stringent handling requirements than might be found for urinary catheters and laparascopic catheters. Many of these types of requirements will be required in the development of tools for minimally invasive surgery. Functionality of the device will define the design requirements. Blood contacting catheters will be used as an example of functionality requirements. A multiplicity of requirements becomes evident as they not only contact blood but also have soft tissue and percutaneous (through the skin) requirements.

Table 1.1. Materials selection guide

Identify

- Predicate devices
- Corporate/institutional predicate devices, testing and regulatory approvals (510(k)s, PMA's, and NDAs)
- Corporate/institutional guidelines, procedures and protocols
- FDA guidelines, CEN guidelines, and standards (ASTM, ANSI, ISO)
- Corporate/institutional R&D reports
- Materials, uses, properties, ASTM and ISO standards

Develop an approach for selection and testing

Table 1.2. Device design and testing as function of materials evaluation

Device Functional Requirements
Prioritization of Requirements
Brain Storming
Medical literature and patents   Nonmedical literature and patents
Networking
Design Approaches
Predicate Devices and Literature—Materials and Failure Modes
Corporate/Institutional 510(k)s, PMA's, and NDA's
Identification of Relevant Standards and Guidelines for Devices, Materials, and Test Methods[1,2]
Corporate/institutional guidelines, protocols, and master files
Regulatory: FDA, CEN
Standards organizations: ISO, ANSI, AAMI, ASTM
Materials Selection:
Requirements
Mechanical, physiochemical, surface, durability, biostability, biocompatibility and thromboresistance[2]
Approach 1   Approach 2   Approach 3   Approach 4
Prototype Component Modeling and Testing Feasibility
New materials and processes — yes
Existing data — no
Determine Sterilization Methods and Test Sterilized Devices and Components
Biocompatibility Screening[3]
Biostability Screening[4]
New technology/application — yes
Bench test
Animal feasibility for efficacy and explant analysis
-- Device analysis: physical and surface
-- Tissue histopathology
Revise Design
Review Functional Requirements
Delineate Potential Failure Modes (Failure Modes and Effects Analysis,—FMEA)
Final Design
Modeling and Testing of Components and Device
- Material qualification—chemical, biocompatibility
- Bench testing—mechanical, durability/fatigue, physiochemical(leachables, permeability, lubricity, etc.)

Implement Biocompatibility Testing
FDA Blue Book Use of ISO=10933 Biological Evaluation of Medical Devices Part 1 and FDA Biocompatibility Flow Chart for Selection of Toxicity Tests for 510(k)s[5,6]

continued on next page

Table 1.2. continued

Shelf-Life Testing
Carcinongenicity Testing for Permanent Implant Devices
Preclinical Efficacy and Safety Testing (Regulatory Guidelines)
Device animal implantation for function and durability
Efficacy measure, e.g., repair, functional measurement
-- In vivo methods—radiology, NMR, Echo, nuclear medicine, assays of blood
-- Explant analysis
-- Device analysis: physical and surface
-- Tissue histopathology
Clinical Evaluation (Regulatory Guidelines)

[1]Table 1.3 Device Guideline Table
[2]Table 1.5 Biomaterials and Properties
[3]Table 1.6 Overview of Screening for Cytotoxicity, Mutagenicity, and Biostability
[4]Table 1.6 Overview of Screening for Cytotoxicity, Mutagenicity, and Biostability
[5]Table 1.6 Overview of Screening for Cytotoxicity, Mutagenicity, and Biostability
[6] Useful for assessing new materials for all biocompatibility evaluations including IDEs/PMAs

Blood contacting catheters have the following general requirements that relate to technique and physiologic interactions:

- Potential damage to the blood vessel which can result in thrombosis and hyperplastic responses. Insertion technique can strongly influence damage.
- Proper sizing of catheter in relation to blood vessel, damage to vessel, flow rate over catheter, more turbulent or static areas can result in thrombosis
- Duration of catheterization—risk of thrombosis and in particular infection increases with time

Catheter Physio-Chemical Properties:

- Physical properties
- Longitudinal stiffness (stiff materials can pierce the vessel wall or damage the vessel wall; vessel wall damage can result in thrombosis)/pushability of catheter
- Torquability of catheter (ability to rotate the catheter)
- Kink resistance
- Memory of preformed curves after insertion
- Burst strength
- Softening of the catheter due to water uptake and warming
- Surface chemistry and effect on blood-materials interaction
- Roughness, pits, and fissures which can result in a nidus of thrombus
- Toxic leachables
- Degradation resulting in toxic leachables and loss of mechanical properties
- Lubricity—drag of catheter could damage tissue
- Effect of manufacturing process on physical and biologic properties
- Sterilization methods—change in mechanical properties, degradation, and toxic leachables
- Coatings: Antithrombotic, Antimicrobial, and Lubricious. Lubricious coatings can have an important role in making the catheter easier to insert and pass over obstructive plaques. However, slippery coatings at the sites the clinician handles the catheter can make them difficult to use.

There are a variety of different blood contacting catheters whose properties and requirements are a function of the specific application.

Table 1.3. Device guideline table

Device	Materials of Construction: Predicate Devices and Corporate Devices/Bill of Materials	Materials Related Design Issues	Standards/Guidelines FDA	Standards/Guidelines ASTM, ANSI, Guidances for Cardio-pulmonary Bypass Oxygenators 510(k) Submissions	Standards/Guidelines ISO
General Biomaterials Standards		Biocompatibility; Additives; Animal evaluation; Sterilization; Shelf-life; Material qualification	Blue Book:95-1: Use of International Standard ISO-10933, "Biological Evaluation of Medical devices Part 1: Evaluation and Testing; Color Additive Status List (Inspection Operations Manual); Shelf Life of Medical devices; Appendix 6, Color Additive for Medical Devices, Pre-Market Approval Manual, Jan. 1998. Deciding When to Submit a 510(k) for a Change to an Existing Device:510(k) Memorandum #K97-1: January 10, 1997; Guidance for FDA Reviewers and Industry—Medical Devices Containing Materials Derived from Animal Sources (Except for In Vitro Diagnostic Devices); Extraction Guidance for	ANSI/AAMI HE48-1993 Human Factors Engineering Guidelines and Preferred Practices for the Design of Medical devices; ANSI/AAMI/ISO 10993-1-1994 Biological Evaluation of Medical devices—Parts 1 - 13 and 16 (see Standards/Guidelines ISO)	ISO-10933 series of Biocompatibility Testing- Part 1: Guidance on selection of tests; Part 2: Animal welfare requirements; Part 3: Tests for genotoxicity, carcinogenicity and reproductive toxicity ; Part 4: Selection of tests for interactions with blood; Part 5: Test for Cytotoxicity: In Vitro Methods; Part 6 Tests for local effects after implantation; Part 7 Ethylene Oxide sterilization residues; Part 8 : Clinical Investigation; Part 9 Degradation of materials related to biological testing; Part 10: Tests for Irritation and Sensitization; -

Table 1.3. continued

Device	Materials of Construction: Predicate Devices and Corporate Devices/Bill of Materials	Materials Related Design Issues	Standards/Guidelines FDA	Standards/Guidelines ASTM, ANSI	Standards/Guidelines ISO
			Polymeric Materials; Draft: A Primer on Medical Device Interactions with Magnetic Resonance Imaging Systems	F1855-98 Standard Specification for Polyoxymethylene (Acetal) for Medical Applications	
				F763 Short-Term Screening of Implant Materials; ASTM: F763 Short-Term Screening of Implant Materials; F748 Selecting Generic Biological Test Methods for Materials and Devices	Sensitization Part 11: Tests for systemic toxicity; Part 12: Sample preparation and reference materials; Part 13: Identification and quantification of degradation products from polymeric medical devices; Part 16: Toxicokinetic study design for degradation products and leachables
				F749 Evaluating Material Extracts by Intracutaneous Injection in the Rabbit; F750 Evaluating Material Extracts by Systemic Injection in the Mouse; F756 Assessment of Hemolytic Properties of Materials; F763 Short-Term Screening of Implant Materials	ISO/DIS 12891-1 Retrieval and analysis of implantable medical devices—Part 1: Retrieval and handling; SO/DIS 14630 Nonactive surgical implants—General requirements; ISO/TR 14283:1995 Implants for surgery—Fundamental principles

Table 1.3. continued

Device	Materials of Construction: Predicate Devices and Corporate Devices/Bill of Materials	Materials Related Design Issues	Standards/Guidelines FDA	Standards/Guidelines ASTM, ANSI	Standards/Guidelines ISO
				F813 Direct Contact Cell Culture Evaluation of Materials for Medical Devices; F1408 Subcutaneous Screening Test for Implant Materials; F1439 Performance of Lifetime Bioassay for the Tumorigenic Potential of Implant Materials; F719 Testing Biomaterials in Rabbits for Primary Skin Irritation; F1251 Polymeric Biomaterials in Medical and Surgical Devices; F604 Silicone Elastomers Used in Medical Applications; F619 Extraction of Medical Plastics; F665 Vinyl Chloride Plastics Used in Biomedical Application; F624 Evaluation of Thermoplastic Polyurethane Solids and Solutions for Biomedical Applications; F639-98a Polyethylene Plastics for Medical Applications; F755 Selection of Porous Polyethylene for Use in Surgical Implants	ISO 15374:1998 Implants for surgery—Requirements for production of forgings; ISO 14630:1997 Nonactive surgical implants—General requirements; ISO 12891-1:1998 Retrieval and analysis of surgical implants—Part 1: Retrieval and handling

Table 1.3. continued

Device	Materials of Construction: Predicate Devices and Corporate Devices/Bill of Materials	Materials Related Design Issues	Standards/Guidelines FDA	Standards/Guidelines ASTM, ANSI	Standards/Guidelines ISO
				F749-98 Standard Practice for Evaluating Material Extracts by Intracutaneous Injection in the Rabbit; F748-98 Standard Practice for Selecting Generic Biological Test Methods for Materials and Devices F665-98 Standard Classification for Vinyl Chloride Plastics Used in Biomedical Application; F648-98 Standard Specification for Ultra-High-Molecular-Weight Polyethylene Powder and Fabricated Form for Surgical Implants; F602-98a Standard Criteria for Implantable Thermoset Epoxy Plastics F640 Radiopacity of Plastics for Medical Use; F641-98a Implantable Epoxy Electronic Encapsulants; F702-98a Polysulfone Resin for Medical Applications; F997-98a Polycarbonate Resin for Medical Applications;	

Table 1.3. continued

Device	Materials of Construction: Predicate Devices and Corporate Devices/Bill of Materials	Materials Related Design Issues	Standards/Guidelines FDA	Standards/Guidelines ASTM, ANSI	Standards/Guidelines CEN
				F1905-98 Standard Practice for Selecting Tests for Determining the Propensity of Materials to Cause Immunotoxicity; F1904-98 Standard Practice for Testing the Biological Responses to Particles In Vivo; F1903-98 Standard Practice for Testing for Biological Responses to Particles In Vitro; F1876-98 Standard Specification for Polyetherketoneetherketoneketone (PEKEKK) Resins for Surgical Implant Applications F1408-97 Standard Practice for Subcutaneous Screening Test for Implant Materials; D3296-98 Standard Specification for FEP-Fluorocarbon TubeF1579 Polyaryletherketone (PAEK) Resins for Surgical Implant Applications; F754 Implantable Polytetrafluoroethylene (PTFE) Polymer Fabricated in Sheet, Tube, and Rod Shapes; Metals and Alloys are listed below under	

Table 1.3. continued

Device	Materials of Construction: Predicate Devices and Corporate Devices/Bill of Materials	Materials Related Design Issues	Standards/Guidelines FDA	Standards/Guidelines ASTM, ANSI	Standards/Guidelines ISO
				Orthopedic and Dental Devices; F560-98 Standard Specification for Unalloyed Tantalum for Surgical Implant Applications	
Cardiovascular		Eficacy; Thrombus; Emboli; Tissue overgrowth, hyperplasia, hemolysis			
Heart Valves		Fatigue and fracture toughness of structural components; Corrosion of metallic components; Sewing cuff—fabric Strength; Fabric porosity; Device compliance; Suturability; Suture retention; Ingrowth of tissue	Draft Replacement Heart Valves—Guidance for Data to be submitted to the FDA in Support of Applications for Premarket Approval and Addendum; Analysis of Explanted Heart Valves		ISO/DIS 5840 Cardiovascular implants—Cardiac valve prostheses

Table 1.3. continued

Device	Materials of Construction: Predicate Devices and Corporate Devices/Bill of Materials	Materials Related Design Issues	Standards/Guidelines FDA	Standards/Guidelines ASTM, ANSI	Standards/Guidelines ISO
Mechanical Heart Valve	Pyrolytic Carbon - housing and bileaflets; Pyrolytic Carbon monoleaflet or bileaflets and metallic housing	Cavitation erosion		ASTM: G32 Cavitation Erosion Using Vibratory Apparatus	
Biologic Heart Valve	Porcine Valve—Stentless	Calcification; Biodegradation; Degree of cross-linking; Shrink temperature			
	Porcine Valve—Stentless; Stented porcine—metallic or plastic	Creep of plastic stent			
	Pericardial valve—metallic or plastic stent	Creep of plastic stent			
Allograft Heart Valve	Human cryopreserved heart valves	Viral contamination	FDA Draft Guidance		

Table 1.3. continued

Device	Materials of Construction: Predicate Devices and Corporate Devices/Bill of Materials	Materials Related Design Issues	Standards/Guidelines FDA	Standards/Guidelines ASTM, ANSI	Standards/Guidelines ISO
Annuloplasty Rings	Polyester Fabric; Titanium; Silicone	Fabric strength; Fabric porosity; Device compliance; Suturability; Suture retention; Ingrowth of Tissue			
Vascular Graft		Biostability; Life testing; Dilatation; Burst Strength	Guidance: Vascular graft manufacturer, Developer, or Representative (Letter); Draft Guidance for the Preparation of Research and Marketing Applications for Vascular graft Prostheses and Cover Letter	ANSI/AAMI VP20-1994 Vascular graft Prostheses;	ISO 7198:1998 Cardiovascular implants—Tubular vascular prostheses
Elastomeric Vascular Graft	Polyurethane	Molecular weight distribution; Porosity—Degree of tissue ingrowth			
Textile Vascular Graft	Polyester: knit, knitted velour,	Molecular weight distribution;			

Table 1.3. continued

Device	Materials of Construction: Predicate Devices and Corporate Devices/Bill of Materials	Materials Related Design Issues	Standards/Guidelines FDA	Standards/Guidelines ASTM, ANSI	Standards/Guidelines ISO
	woven, woven velour, pre- coated (e.g., aldehyde cross-linked collagen, gelatin, albumin to prevent need for pre-clotting).	Porosity—flow rate of water at physiologic pressure; Ability to pre-clot			
Expanded PTFE	Polytetraflouroethylene (PTFE): with or without external PTFE wrap	Thermal analysis to determine % sintering; Internodal distance as measure of porosity			
Bioprosthetic—**Bovine; Porcine Vascular Graft**		Degree of cross-linking; Shrink temperature; Calcification			
Allograft **Vascular Graft**	Human cryopreserved femoral, iliac, and aortic vessels	Cryopreservation technique; Viral contamination			
Cardiology Catheters	Polyolefin, Polyamide,	Trackability; Torquabilty;	Guidance for the Submission of Research		ISO/DIS 10555-2 Sterile, single-use intravascular catheters—Part 2: Angiographic catheters

Table 1.3. continued

Device	Materials of Construction: Predicate Devices and Corporate Devices/Bill of Materials	Materials Related Design Issues	Standards/Guidelines FDA	Standards/Guidelines ASTM, ANSI	Standards/Guidelines ISO
	Polyamide elastomer, Polyester, Metallic, or Composite shaft; Heparin Coatings	Lubricity; Stiffness; Burst strength of catheter and balloon; Thrombogenicity; Characterization of shaft by thermal and mechanical analysis	and Marketing Applications for Interventional Cardiology Devices—PTCA Catheters, Atherectomy Catheters, Lasers, Intravascular Stents		
Angioplasty Catheters	Compliant (polyolefin or polyamide) or noncompliant (polyester) balloon	Characterization of balloon by thermal and mechanical analysis; Degree of crystallinity; burst strength; toughness; Modulus of balloon material	PTCA Catheter System Testing Guidance for the Submission of an IDE Application and a PMA Application		ISO/DIS 10555-4 Sterile, single-use intravascular catheters—Part 4: Balloon dilatation catheters
	Laser, Atherectomy		FDA Guidelines for the Preparation and Contents of an IDE Applications for Laser Devices Used in the Treatment of Atherosclerotic Disease		

Table 1.3. continued

Device	Materials of Construction: Predicate Devices and Corporate Devices/Bill of Materials	Materials Related Design Issues	Standards/Guidelines FDA	Standards/Guidelines ASTM, ANSI	Standards/Guidelines ISO
Vavluloplasty Catheters	Compliant (polyolefin or polyamide) or noncompliant (polyester) balloon	Characterization of balloon by thermal and mechanical analysis; Degree of crystallinity; burst strength; toughness; Modulus of balloon material	FDA Balloon Valvuloplasty Guidance for the Submission of an IDE Application and a PMA Applications		
Pacemaker Leads	Polyurethane; Silicone	Biostability of polyurethane in presence of corrosion by-products; Water absorption; Insulating properties	FDA Implantable Pacemaker Lead Testing Guidance for the Submission of a Section 510K Notification		
Endovascular Stent	Heparin coatings, incorporation of antirestenotic agents	Biostability; Corrosion; Life testing; Dilatation; Burst strength; Vessel recoil after ballooning and stent placement; Thrombogenicity	Guidance for the Submission of Research and Marketing Applications for Interventional Cardiology Devices—PTCA Catheters, Atherectormy Catheters,		

Table 1.3. continued

Device	Materials of Construction: Predicate Devices and Corporate Devices/Bill of Materials	Materials Related Design Issues	Standards/Guidelines FDA	Standards/Guidelines ASTM, ANSI	Standards/Guidelines ISO
		and Hyperplastic/ Restenotic response	Lasers, intravascular stents; carotid stent—Suggestions for content of submissions to the FDA in support of investigational device exemption (IDE) applications		
	Self expanding stents (Cobalt-Cr alloys; Nitinol memory/ superelastic alloys)	Force of self expansion			
	Balloon expandable stents (tantalum, stainless steel, Nitinol)	Force to balloon expand			
Circulatory Assist Devices		Durability; Biostability; Fatigue and fracture toughness of structural components;			

Table 1.3. continued

Device	Materials of Construction: Predicate Devices and Corporate Devices/Bill of Materials	Materials Related Design Issues	Standards/Guidelines FDA	Standards/Guidelines ASTM, ANSI	Standards/Guidelines ISO
		Corrosion of metallic components			
Intraaortic Balloon Pumps	Polyurethane elastomer balloon	Creep of balloon; Characterization of balloon by thermal and mechanical analysis; Burst strength; Toughness; Trackability; Torquabilty; Lubricity; Stiffness; Burst strength of catheter and balloon; Thrombogenicity; Characterization of shaft by thermal and mechanical analysis	Determining equivalence of intraaortic balloon catheters under the 510 K regulation		
Centrifugal Pumps	Plastic housings and impeller (polycarbonate; acrylics) or titanium alloy impeller	Bearing effect on blood element destruction			

Table 1.3. continued

Device	Materials of Construction: Predicate Devices and Corporate Devices/Bill of Materials	Materials Related Design Issues	Standards/Guidelines FDA	Standards/Guidelines ASTM, ANSI	Standards/Guidelines ISO
Left Ventricular and Total Artificial Heart Devices—Vascular Graft Components, Heart Valve Components.	Polyurethane Pumping surfaces, Textured Polyurethane Pumping Surfaces, Polyolefin Rubber, Gelatin Coatings, Titanium Housing, Engineering plastic housing, e.g., Polysulfone, carbon fiber reinforced polysulfone; Textured blood contact surfaces.	Creep of pumping surface; Characterization of bladder by thermal and mechanical analysis; toughness; tear resistance; calcification; infection	FDA Guidance for the Preparation and Content of Applications to the FDA for Ventricular Assist and Total Artificial Hearts		
Hemodialyzers Peritoneal Dialysis	Cellulosics; polycarbonate, polysulfone, polyacrylonitrile sodium methallylsulfonate	Water permeability, pore size, molecular weight cut-off	Guidelines for Premarket Testing of New Conventional Hemodialyzers, High Permeability hemodialyzers, and Hemofilters	ANSI/AAMI RD17-1994 Hemodialyzer Blood Tubing; ANSI/AAMI BF7-1989 Blood Transfusion Micro-Filters	ISO/DIS 7199 Cardiovascular implants and artificial organs—Blood-gas exchangers; ISO 8637:1989 Hemodialysers, hemofilters and hemoconcentrators; ISO 8638:1989 Extracorporeal blood circuit for hemodialysers, hemofilters and hemoconcentrators;

Table 1.3. continued

Device	Materials of Construction: Predicate Devices and Corporate Devices/Bill of Materials	Materials Related Design Issues	Standards/Guidelines FDA	Standards/Guidelines ASTM, ANSI	Standards/Guidelines ISO
Oxygenators and In-Line Filters	Silicone; microporous polypropylene; polysulfone	Oxygen and carbon dioxide permeation; pore size	FDA Guidance for Safety and Effectiveness Data Required in Premarket Notification (510K) Applications for Blood Oxygenators; Guidance for the Submission of 510(k) Premarket Notifications for Cardiovascular Intravascular Filters—Version 1.0		
Intravenous Catheters	Polyolefin, Polyurethane, PVC IV catheters; Heparin coatings; Incorporation of antimicrobial agents	Ease of insertion; Lubricity; Stiffness; Burst strength of catheter; Thrombogenicity; Bacterial adherence	Catheter Guidance; Guidance on Premarket Notification (510K) Submission for Short-term and Long-term Intravascular Catheters		ISO 10555-1:1995 Sterile, single-use intravascular catheters—Part 1: General requirements
Central Venous Catheters	Heparin Coatings	Ease of insertion; Lubricity; Stiffness; Burst strength of catheter;	Guidance on Premarket Notification (510K) Submission for Short-term and Long-term Intravascular Catheters		ISO/DIS 10555-3 Sterile, single-use intravascular catheters—Part 3: Central venous catheters

Table 1.3. continued

Device	Materials of Construction: Predicate Devices and Corporate Devices/Bill of Materials	Materials Related Design Issues	Standards/Guidelines FDA	Standards/Guidelines ASTM, ANSI	Standards/Guidelines ISO
		Thrombogenicity; Tissue overgrowth; Fibrous sheath formation over length of catheter; Water absorption; softening; Bacterial adherence; Resistance to infection			
Acute	Polyolefin, Polyurethane, PVC CVC catheters; Incorporation of antimicrobial agents				
Chronic	Silicone or Polyurethane shafts; Incorporation of antimicrobial agents on shaft; polyester cuff for tissue ingrowth; degradable cuff with antimicrobial agents				

Table 1.3. continued

Device	Materials of Construction: Predicate Devices and Corporate Devices/Bill of Materials	Materials Related Design Issues	Standards/Guidelines FDA	Standards/Guidelines ASTM, ANSI	Standards/Guidelines ISO
Implantable Central Venous Ports	Silicone, Polyurethane catheters; Titanium or stainless steel ports; silicone rubber septum	Ease of insertion; Lubricity; Stiffness; Burst strength of catheter; Thrombogenicity; Bacterial adherence; Fibrous tissue formation around port; Multiple needle penetrations of port	Guidance on 510K Submission for Implanted Infusion Ports		
Soft Tissue (Implants, Reconstruction, Catheters, Ocular; Wound Dressings, Esophageal and Tracheal Prostheses, Biliary Prostheses and Skin Contact)		Efficacy; Wound healing, Biocompatibility; Fibrous tissue formation; Fibrous tissue contracture; Tissue adhesion; Infection; Hypersensitivity; Tissue erosion	Guidance for Industry; Guidance for the Content of Premarket Notifications for Esophageal and Tracheal Prostheses; Guidance for the Content of Premarket Notifications for Metal Expandable Biliary Stents; Protocol for Dermal Toxicity Testing for Medical devices in Contact with Skin (Reformatted 12/17/97)	F1441-92(1998) Standard Specification for Soft-Tissue Expander Devices	

Table 1.3. continued

Device	Materials of Construction: Predicate Devices and Corporate Devices/Bill of Materials	Materials Related Design Issues	Standards/Guidelines FDA	Standards/Guidelines ASTM, ANSI	Standards/Guidelines ISO
Urologic Implants and Devices: Urinary Incontinence	Collagen injections; PTFE dispersions; Silicone devices	Tissue irritation; Bulking effect; Tissue erosion; Bacterial adherence and resistance to infection	Draft Guidance for Preparation of PMA Applications for the Implanted Mechanical/ Hydraulic Urinary continence Device; Draft Guidance for Preclinical and Clinical Investigations of Urethral Bulking Agents Used in the Treatment of Urinary Incontinence		
Urologic Implants and Devices: Benign Prostatic Hyperplasia; Ureteral Strictures	Compliant (polyolefin or polyamide) or noncompliant (polyester) balloon; Self expanding stents (Cobalt-Cr alloys; Nitinol memory/ superelastic alloys) or balloon expandable stents (stainless steel,	Recoil after ballooning or stent placement; Tissue thickening after ballooning or stent placement; Tissue erosion with stent	Draft Guidance for Clinical Investigations of Devices Used for the Treatment of Benign Prostatic Hyperplasia (BPH); Draft Guidance for the Content of Premarket Notification for Urologic Balloon Dilation Catheters;		

Table 1.3. continued

Device	Materials of Construction: Predicate Devices and Corporate Devices/Bill of Materials	Materials Related Design Issues	Standards/Guidelines FDA	Standards/Guidelines ASTM, ANSI	Standards/Guidelines ISO
	titanium)		Guidance for the Content of Premarket Notifications for Ureteral Stents		
Testicular and Penile Implants	Silicone elastomer; Silicone gel; Silicone gel substitutes	Tissue inflammation; fibrous capsule contracture; Rupture of shell; Tissue adhesion; Migration of device; Tissue erosion; Matching compliance of surrounding soft tissue; gel leakage	Guidance to Manufacturers on the Development of Required Postapproval Epidemiologic Study Protocols for Testicular Implants; Draft Guidance for Preparation of PMA Application for Testicular Prostheses; Draft Guidelines for Preparation of PMA Applications for Penile Inflatable Implants; Draft Guidance for the Content for Premarket Notifications for Penile Rigidity Implants		
Urinary Catheters	Silicone; Latex; Antimicrobial	Lubricity; Bacterial Adherence;	Guidance of Premarket Notifications for Conventional and	ASTM: F623 Foley Catheter	

Table 1.3. continued

Device	Materials of Construction: Predicate Devices and Corporate Devices/Bill of Materials	Materials Related Design Issues	Standards/Guidelines FDA	Standards/Guidelines ASTM, ANSI	Standards/Guidelines ISO
	coatings	Resistance to infection; Calcium deposits in long term use	Antimicrobial Foley Catheters; Guidance to Manufacturers on the Development of Required Postapproval		
Laparoscopic Catheters, Gynecologic Devices	Metallic or engineering plastic shafts	Lubricity; Ease of use	Hyterscopes and Laparascopes, Insufflators and Other Related Instrumentations: Submission Requirements for a 510K; SE Comparison Chart for Laparoscopes; Guidance (Guidelines) for Evaluation of Tubal Occlusion Devices; Hysteroscopic and Laparoscopic Insufflators: Submission Guidance for a 510K;		
Antiadhesion Barriers	Hydrogels; Hyaluoranic acid; Cellulosics; Collagen	Degree of tissue adhesion; Lack of inflammatory response during resorption and tissue healing	Guidance for Absorbable Adhesion Barrier Devices used in Abdominal and/ or Pelvic Surgery		

Table 1.3. continued

Device	Materials of Construction: Predicate Devices and Corporate Devices/Bill of Materials	Materials Related Design Issues	Standards/Guidelines FDA	Standards/Guidelines ASTM, ANSI	Standards/Guidelines ISO
Neurologic Devices			Guidance on Biocompatibility Requirements for Long Term Neurological Implants: Part 3—Implant Model	NSI/AAMI NS15-1995 : Implantable Peripheral Nerve Stimulators	
Hydrocephalus Shunts	Silicone	Protein deposition; Freedom from occlusion; Tissue overgrowth—neural tissue brain side, thrombus; tissue overgrowth on venous/peritoneal side		ASTM: F647 Evaluating and Specifying Implantable Shunt Assemblies for Neurosurgical Application	SO 7197:1989 Neurosurgical implants—Sterile, single-use hydrocephalus shunts and components
Clips		Corrosion; Neural tissue compatibility		F1542 the Requirements and Disclosure of Self-Closing Aneurysm Clips	ISO 9713:1990 Neurosurgical implants—Self-closing intracranial aneurysm clips
Reconstructive Surgery		Biostability; Tissue inflammation		ASTM: F881 Silicone Elastomer Facial Implants; F981 Assessment of Compatibility of Biomaterials for Surgical Implants with Respect to Effect of Materials on	

Table 1.3. continued

Device	Materials of Construction: Predicate Devices and Corporate Devices/Bill of Materials	Materials Related Design Issues	Standards/Guidelines FDA	Standards/Guidelines ASTM, ANSI	Standards/Guidelines ISO
				Muscle and Bone; F622 Preformed Cranioplasty Plates that Can be Altered	
Mammary Prostheses—Silicone Gel Filled	Silicone elastomer; Polyurethane; Silicone gel; Texture surfaces; Permeation barrier to silicone gel	Tissue inflammation; fibrous capsule contracture; Rupture of shell; Tissue adhesion; Migration of device; Tissue erosion; Matching compliance of surrounding soft tissue; Leakage of gel	Draft Guidance Preparation of FDA Submissions of Silicone Gel-Filled Breast Prostheses, Oct. 1999		
Nonsilicone Gel Filled	Hydrogels; Saline	Deflation; Permeation of gel through shell; Tissue inflammation; fibrous capsule contracture; Rupture of shell; Tissue adhesion; Migration of device; Tissue erosion; Matching	Draft Guidance for Preparation of PMA Applications for Silicone Inflatable (Saline) Breast Prosthesis; Draft Guidance for Testing of Alternative Breast Prostheses (nonsilicone gel filled)		

Table 1.3. continued

Device	Materials of Construction: Predicate Devices and Corporate Devices/Bill of Materials	Materials Related Design Issues	Standards/Guidelines FDA	Standards/Guidelines ASTM, ANSI	Standards/Guidelines ISO
		compliance of surrounding soft tissue			
Patches—	Bioprosthetic Bovine Pericardial Human Dura mater	Calcification; Immune responses; Viral contamination	FDA Guidance for 510K Review of Processed Human Dura Mater		
Wound Dressing		Water and oxygen permeability; Adhesion to wound bed; Flexibility and conformability; permeation of antibiotics; Resistance to infection; Ease of removal; Enhancement of epidermal regeneration; Suitability for server burns and ulcers	Checklists for Wound Dressing 510K Interactive Wound and Burn Dressing IDE Submission; Draft Guidance for the Preparation of a Premarket Notification for a Non-Interactive Wound and Burn Dressing		

Table 1.3. continued

Device	Materials of Construction: Predicate Devices and Corporate Devices/Bill of Materials	Materials Related Design Issues	Standards/Guidelines FDA	Standards/Guidelines ASTM, ANSI	Standards/Guidelines ISO
	Synthetic; Bioprosthetic; Active; Allograft; Biohybrid	Viral contamination in allografts; Tissue irritants in bioprosthetics; Cryopreservation technique for allograft; Cell viability, health and contamination in biohybrid			
Medical Gloves & Oral Facial Prosthetic Devices	Latex, vinyl; polyurethane	Skin irritation; Leachables; hypersensitivity; Feel through glove; Tear resistance	Interim Guidance on Protein Content Labeling for Latex Medical Gloves (with cover letter to medical glove manufacturers); Submissions for Testing for Skin Sensitizating to Chemicals in Latex Medical Products	ASTM: D3577 Rubber Surgical Gloves; D3578 Rubber Examination Gloves; D3579 Rubber Surgical Drainage Tubes, Penrose-Type; D3738 Rubber-Coated Cloth Hospital Sheeting; D3772 Rubber Finger Cots; D5151 Detection of Holes in Medical Gloves; D5250 Poly(vinyl chloride) Gloves for Medical Application; F1027 Assessment of Tissue and Cell Compatibility of Orofacial Prosthetic Materials and Devices	

Table 1.3. continued

Device	Materials of Construction: Predicate Devices and Corporate Devices/Bill of Materials	Materials Related Design Issues	Standards/Guidelines FDA	Standards/Guidelines ASTM, ANSI	Standards/Guidelines ISO
Contact Lenses	Acrylics; Hydrogels; Silicone copolymers	Oxygen permeability; Resistance to infection; Epidermal cell irritation adhesion; Optical parameters; UV absorption			ISO/DIS 9339-1 Optics and optical instruments—Contact lenses—Determination of the thickness—Part 1: Rigid contact lenses; ISO/DIS 9340 Optics and optical instruments—Contact lenses—Determination of strains; ISO/DIS 9341 Optics and optical Instruments—Contact lenses—Determination of inclusions and surface imperfections of rigid contact lenses; ISO 9363-1:1994 Optics and optical instruments—Contact lenses—Determination of cytotoxicity of contact lens material—Part 1: Agaroverlay test and growth inhibition test; ISO 9394:1994 Optics and optical instruments—Determination of biological compatibility of contact lens material—Testing of the contact lens system by ocular study with rabbit eyes; ISO/DIS 9913-1 Optics and optical instruments—Contact lenses—Determination of oxygen

Table 1.3. continued

Device	Materials of Construction: Predicate Devices and Corporate Devices/Bill of Materials	Materials Related Design Issues	Standards/Guidelines FDA	Standards/Guidelines ASTM, ANSI	Standards/Guidelines ISO
					permeability and transmissibility with the FATT method; ISO/DIS 10339 Optics and optical instruments—Contact lenses Determination of water content of soft lenses; ISO 10340:1995 Optics and optical instruments—Contact lenses — Method for determining the extractable substances; ISO/DIS 11980 Optics and optical instruments—Contact lenses and contact lens care products—Guidelines for clinical investigations; ISO/DIS 11981 Optics and optical instruments—Contact lenses and contact lens care products—Methods for the determination of the physical compatibility of contact lenses with contact lens care products; ISO/DIS 11985 Optics and optical instruments—Contact lenses Ageing by UV and visible radiation (in vitro method); ISO/DIS 11986 Optics and optical instruments—Contact lenses and contact lens care products—Test

Table 1.3. continued

Device	Materials of Construction: Predicate Devices and Corporate Devices/Bill of Materials	Materials Related Design Issues	Standards/Guidelines FDA	Standards/Guidelines ASTM, ANSI	Standards/Guidelines ISO
					methods for preservative uptake and release; ISO/DIS 11987 Optics and optical instruments Contact lenses—Methods for the determination of shelf-life; ISO/DIS 13212 Optics and optical instruments—Contact lenses and contact lens care products—Test methods for the determination of shelf-life and in-use stability; ISO/DIS 14534 Optics and optical instruments—Contact lenses and contact lens care products—Fundamental requirements
Intraocular Lenses	Acrylics; Silicone copolymers	Oxygen permeability, Optical parameters; Leachables, tissue irritation; Cell adhesion; Flexibility	Guidance Document Multifocal Intraocular Lens IDEs: Preclinical and Clinical Uses; New Requirements for Investigations of Anterior Chamber Intraocular Lenses (IOL); Guidelines for Intraocular Lenses		ISO/DIS 11979-3 Optics and optical instruments—Intraocular lenses—Part 3: Mechanical properties and their test methods; ISO/DIS 11979-5 Optics and optical instruments—Intraocular lenses—Part 5: Biocompatibility

Table 1.3. continued

Device	Materials of Construction: Predicate Devices and Corporate Devices/Bill of Materials	Materials Related Design Issues	Standards/Guidelines FDA	Standards/Guidelines ASTM, ANSI	Standards/Guidelines ISO
			Guidance Document Approval Requirements for IOLs with an Extended Power Range		
Cochlear Implants	Electrode and insulation material; Engineering plastic housing or metallic alloy housing	Soft and hard tissue compatibility; Chronic tissue irritation of soft tissue and adhacent nerves	Guidance for the Arrangement and Content of a Premarket Approval (PMA) Application for a Cochlear Implant in Children Ages 2 through 17 Years; Guidance for the Arrangement and Content of a Premarket Approval (PMA) Application for a Cochlear Implant in Children Adults at Least 18 years of age.		
Cells to Produce Biologic	Seeded on synthetic	Purity of cell type, viability, viral	Points to Consider in the Characterization of Cell Line Used to Produce Biological Products		

Table 1.3. continued

Device	Materials of Construction: Predicate Devices and Corporate Devices/Bill of Materials	Materials Related Design Issues	Standards/Guidelines FDA	Standards/Guidelines ASTM, ANSI	Standards/Guidelines ISO
Products	and bioprosthetics substrate; Degradable polymers; Protein and peptide cell adhesion agents	contamination; compatibility with host (autologous cells versus allograft versus xenograft)			
Hard Tissue		Efficacy; Bone formation; Bone resorption; Infection; Sclerotic bone formation; Stress-shielding; Bone adhesion to device; Fibrous tissue formation			
Orthopedic and Joint Prostheses	Stainless steels; Cobalt chrome alloys; Titanium alloys; Calcium phosphate; Hydroxyapatite and bioglass coatings and bone fillers;	Corrosion; Life testing; Stress and fatigue analysis and testing; Wear; Fracture toughness; Biostability; Infection; Resorption/ dissolution rate of	Draft Guidance for the Preparation of Premarket (510K) Applications for Orthopedic Devices—The Basic Elements; Guidance Information on Surface Characteristics of Implant Metals; Guidance Information	ASTM: F1091 Wrought Cobalt-Chromium Alloy Surgical Fixation Wire; F1108 Ti6Al4V Alloy Castings for Surgical Implants; F1058 Wrought Cobalt-Chromium-Nickel-Molybdenum-Iron Alloy for Surgical Implant Applications	ISO/DIS 5832- 1-12 Implants for surgery—Metallic materials; ISO 5839:1985 Implants for surgery—Orthopedic joint prostheses—Basic requirements; ISO 6018:1987 Orthopaedic implants—General requirements for marking, packaging and labeling

Table 1.3. continued

Device	Materials of Construction: Predicate Devices and Corporate Devices/Bill of Materials	Materials Related Design Issues	Standards/Guidelines FDA	Standards/Guidelines ASTM, ANSI	Standards/Guidelines ISO
	Porous coatings	bioactive coating	on Galvanic Corrosion of Implant Metals; Orthopedic		
			Device Approval and Labeling; Guidance Document for Testing Orthopedic Implants with Modified Metallic Surfaces Apposing Bone or Bone Cement; 510(k) Information Needed for Hydroxyapatite Coated Orthopedic Implants	F1295-97a Wrought Titanium-6 Aluminum-7 Niobium Alloy for Surgical Implant Applications; F1314 Wrought Nitrogen Strengthened-22 Chromium-12.5 Nickel-5 Manganese-2.5 Molybdenum Stainless Steel Bar and Wire for Surgical Implants	ISO 6475:1989 Implants for surgery—Metal bone screws with asymmetrical thread and spherical under-surface; ISO 8827:1988 Implants for surgery—Staples with parallel legs for orthopaedic use—General requirements; ISO 9268:1988 Implants for surgery
				F1341 Unalloyed Titanium Wire for Surgical Implant Applications; F1350 Stainless Steel Surgical Fixation Wire; F136-98 Wrought Titanium 6Al-4V ELI Alloy for Surgical Implant Applications; F1377-98a Cobalt-Chromium Molybdenum Powder for Coating of Orthopedic	— Metal bone screws with conical under-surface of head—Dimensions; ISO 9269:1988 Implants for surgery—Metal bone plates—Holes and slots corresponding to screws with conical under-surface;

Table 1.3. continued

Device	Materials of Construction: Predicate Devices and Corporate Devices/Bill of Materials	Materials Related Design Issues	Standards/Guidelines FDA	Standards/Guidelines ASTM, ANSI	Standards/Guidelines ISO
				Implants; F138-97 Stainless Steel Bar and Wire for Surgical Implants (Special Quality); F139 Stainless Steel Sheet and Strip for Surgical Implants (Special Quality)	ISO 10334:1994 Implants for surgery—Malleable wires for use as sutures; ISO/DIS 13782 Implants for surgery—Metallic materials—Unalloyed tantalum for surgical implant applications
				F1472 Wrought TI-6Al-4V Alloy for Surgical Implant Applications; F1537 Wrought Cobalt-28-Chromium-6-Molybdenum Alloy for Surgical Implants; F1579 Polyaryletherketone (PAEK) Resins for Surgical Implant Applications	ISO 5834-2:1998 Implants for surgery—Ultra-high molecular weight polyethylene—Part 2: Moulded forms; ISO 5834-1:1998 Implants for surgery—Ultra-high molecular weight polyethylene—Part 1: Powder form
				F1586 Wrought Nitrogen Strengthened-21 Chromium-10 Nickel-3 Manganese-2.5 Molybdenum Stainless Steel Bar for Surgical Implants; F745 18 Chromium-12.5 Nickel-2.5 Molybdenum Stainless Steel for Cast and Solution-Annealed Surgical Implant Applications	ISO 14602:1998 Nonactive surgical implants—Implants for Osteosynthesis—Particular requirements

Table 1.3. continued

Device	Materials of Construction: Predicate Devices and Corporate Devices/Bill of Materials	Materials Related Design Issues	Standards/Guidelines FDA	Standards/Guidelines ASTM, ANSI	Standards/Guidelines ISO
				F560 Unalloyed Tantalum for Surgical Implant Applications; F561 Analysis of Retrieved Metallic Orthopaedic Implants; F562 Wrought Cobalt-35 Nickel-20 Chromium-10 Molybdenum Alloy for Surgical Implant Applications; F563 Wrought Cobalt-Nickel-Chromium-	
				Molybdenum-Tungsten-Iron Alloy for Surgical Implant Applications; F601 Fluorescent Penetrant Inspection of Metallic Surgical Implants; F629 Radiography of Cast Metallic Surgical Implants	
				F620 Titanium 6Al-4V ELI Alloy Forgings for Surgical Implants; F621 Stainless Steel Forgings for Surgical Implants; F702 Polysulfone Resin for Medical Applications; F75 Cast Cobalt-Chromium-Molybdenum Alloy for Surgical Implant	

Table 1.3. continued

Device	Materials of Construction: Predicate Devices and Corporate Devices/Bill of Materials	Materials Related Design Issues	Standards/Guidelines FDA	Standards/Guidelines ASTM, ANSI	Standards/Guidelines ISO
				Applications F67 Unalloyed Titanium for Surgical Implant Applications; F688 Wrought Cobalt-35 Nickel-20 Chromium-10 Molybdenum Alloy Plate, Sheet, and Foil for Surgical Implants; F961 Cobalt-Nickel-Chromium-Molybdenum Alloy Forgings for Surgical Implant Applications F899 Stainless Steel Billet, Bar, and Wire for Surgical Instruments; F90 Wrought Cobalt-Chromium-Tungsten-Nickel Alloy for Surgical Implant Applications; F799 Cobalt-28Chromium-6Molybdenum Alloy Forgings for Surgical Implants; F1089 Corrosion of Surgical Instruments; F746 Pitting or Crevice Corrosion of Metallic Surgical Implant Materials; F86 Surface Preparation and Marking of Metallic Surgical Implants F1873-98 Standard Specification for High-Purity Dense Yttria	

Table 1.3. continued

Device	Materials of Construction: Predicate Devices and Corporate Devices/Bill of Materials	Materials Related Design Issues	Standards/Guidelines FDA	Standards/Guidelines ASTM, ANSI	Standards/Guidelines ISO
				Tetragonal Zirconium Oxide Polycrystal (Y-TZP) for Surgical Implant Applications; F1813-97 Standard Specification for Wrought Titanium -12 Molybdenum -6 Zirconium -2 Iron Alloy For Surgical Implant Applications; F1801-97 Standard Practice for Corrosion Fatigue Testing of Metallic Implant Materials; F1800-97 Standard Test Method for Cyclic Fatigue Testing of Metal Tibial Tray Components of Total Knee Joint Replacements F983 Permanent Marking of Orthopaedic Implant Components	
Joint Implants	Metallic stems-cemented; porous coated or bioactive coated	Loosening; Wear at joint; Wear debris;	Draft Guidance Document for Femoral Stem Prostheses; Draft Guidance Document for the Testing of Orthopedic Implants with Metallic Plasma	F1044 Shear Testing of Porous Metal Coatings; F1147 Tension Testing of Porous Metal Coatings; F1044 Shear Testing of Porous Metal Coatings; F1147 Tension Testing of Porous Metal Coatings; F1185 Composition of Ceramic	ISO 7206-1-9:1994 Implants for surgery—Partial and total hip joint prostheses—Parts 1- 9; ISO 7207-1:1994 Implants for surgery—Femoral and tibial components for partial and total knee joint prostheses;

Table 1.3. continued

Device	Materials of Construction: Predicate Devices and Corporate Devices/Bill of Materials	Materials Related Design Issues	Standards/Guidelines FDA	Standards/Guidelines ASTM, ANSI	Standards/Guidelines ISO
		Lubicity at joint; Breakdown of cement, porous coating; and bioactive coating; Bone adhesion; Bone resorption; Stress shielding	Sprayed Porous Coatings Subject to Required Post Market Surveillance;	Hydroxylapatite for Surgical Implants	
		Resorption/ dissolution rate of bioactive coating; Cracking and flaking of coating	Draft Guidance for the Preparation of Premarket Notification (510K) for Cemented Semi-Constrained Knee; Calcium Phosphate (Ca-P) Coating Draft Guidance for Preparation of FDA Submissions for Orthopedic and Dental Endosseous Implants	F1223 Determination of Total Knee Replacement Constraint; F1440 Cyclic Fatigue Testing of Metallic Stemmed Hip Arthroplasty Femoral Without Components Torsion;	ISO/TR 9325:1989 Implants for surgery—Partial and total hip joint prostheses—Recommendations for simulators for evaluation of hip joint prostheses; ISO/TR 9326:1989 Implants for surgery—Partial and total hip joint prostheses
				F1814-97a Standard Guide for Evaluating Modular Hip and Knee Joint Components; F1800-97 Standard Test Method for Cyclic Fatigue Testing of Metal	

Table 1.3. continued

Device	Materials of Construction: Predicate Devices and Corporate Devices/Bill of Materials	Materials Related Design Issues	Standards/Guidelines FDA	Standards/Guidelines ASTM, ANSI	Standards/Guidelines ISO
				Tibial Tray Components of Total Knee Joint Replacements; F1875-98 Standard Practice for Fretting Corrosion Testing of Modular Implant Interfaces: Hip Femoral Head-bore and Cone Taper Interface; F1440-92(1997) Standard Practice for Cyclic Fatigue Testing of Metallic Stemmed Hip Arthroplasty Femoral Components Without Torsion	
			Guidance Document for Testing Non-articulating "Mechanically Locked" Modular Implant Components	F732 Reciprocating Pin-on-Flat Evaluation of Friction and Wear Properties of Polymeric Materials for Use in Total Joint Prostheses F1781-97 Standard Specification for Elastomeric Flexible Hinge Finger Total Joint Implants	ISO 9583:1993 Implants for surgery—Nondestructive testing—Liquid penetrant inspection of metallic surgical implants; ISO 9584:1993 Implants for surgery—Nondestructive testing—Radiographic examination of cast metallic surgical implants
	Engineering plastic; Engineering plastic carbon fiber reinforced stem	Stiffness; carbon fiber release and tissue irritation		F1579 Polyaryletherketone (PAEK) Resins for Surgical Implant Applications; F702 Polysulfone Resin for Medical Applications;	

Table 1.3. continued

Device	Materials of Construction: Predicate Devices and Corporate Devices/Bill of Materials	Materials Related Design Issues	Standards/Guidelines FDA	Standards/Guidelines ASTM, ANSI	Standards/Guidelines ISO
	Ceramic head and neck	Fracture toughness of ceramic; high density without voids/	Guidance Document for the Preparation of Premarket Notification for 510k for Ceramic Ball Hip Systems	F603 High-Purity Dense Aluminum Oxide for Surgical Implant Application	ISO 6474:1994 Implants for surgery—Ceramic materials based on high purity alumina; ISO/DIS 13356 Implants for surgery—Ceramic materials based on yttria-stabilized tetragonal zirconia (Y-TZP)
	Acetabular cup: UHMW PE, Ceramic or metallic cup with high wear surface treatment	Micro-wear particles; Creep of UHMW PE; Biostability	Guidance Document for Testing Acetabular Cup Prostheses; Draft Requirements for Ultrahigh Molecular Weight Polytethylene (UHMWPE) Used in Orthopedic Devices		ISO 5834-1—2:1985 Implants for surgery—Ultra-high molecular weight polyethylene—Part 1: Powder form; Part 2: Moulded forms
	Acetabular cup: Cemented, porous coated or bioactive coated			F1044 Shear Testing of Porous Metal Coatings; F1147 Tension Testing of Porous Metal Coatings; F1160 Constant Stress Amplitude Fatigue Testing of Porous Metal-Coated Metallic Materials; F1538 Glass and Glass Ceramic Biomaterials for Implantation	

Table 1.3. continued

Device	Materials of Construction: Predicate Devices and Corporate Devices/Bill of Materials	Materials Related Design Issues	Standards/Guidelines FDA	Standards/Guidelines ASTM, ANSI	Standards/Guidelines ISO
	Bone Cement	Viscosity, heat generation, setting time, Residual monomer and polymerization additives, tissue damage from heat and residuals; particles and wear of acetabular cup	Draft Outline for a Guidance Document for Testing Orthopedic Bone Cement	F451 Acrylic Bone Cement	3:1992 Implants for surgery—Acrylic resin cements
	Porous coating	Degree of porosisty; Corrosion rate for metallics/ Biodegradation nonmetallics; Animal evaluation of bone ingrowth; cracking and flaking of coating		F1044 Shear Testing of Porous Metal Coatings; F1147 Tension Testing of Porous Metal Coatings; F1160 Constant Stress Amplitude Fatigue Testing of Porous Metal-Coated Metallic Materials; F1854-98 Standard Test Method for Stereological Evaluation of Porous Coatings on Medical Implants	
Ligaments	Polyester fabric;	Attachment to bone; bone formation	Guidance Document for the Preparation of IDE and PMA Applications		

Table 1.3. continued

Device	Materials of Construction: Predicate Devices and Corporate Devices/Bill of Materials	Materials Related Design Issues	Standards/Guidelines FDA	Standards/Guidelines ASTM, ANSI	Standards/Guidelines ISO
	Polypropylene fabric; expanded PTFE; bioprosthetic bovine tissue; metallic staples and wire	around attachment in bone; loosening; tearing; wear; tissue ingrowth; calcification	for Intra-Articular Prosthetic Knee Ligament; Guidance Document for Testing Bone Anchor Devices		
Fracture Fixation Devices	Stainless steels; Cobalt chrome alloys; Titanium alloys	Stabilization of bone fracture and bone fragments; stress transfer; Stiffness; Resistance to bending and torsion; Fretting corrosion; stress shielding, bone resorption		F1264 Mechanical Performance Considerations for Intramedullary Fixation Devices; F543 -98 Cortical Bone Screws; F564 Bone Staples	ISO 5835:1991 Implants for surgery—Metal bone screws with hexagonal drive connection, spherical under-surface of head, asymmetrical thread—Dimensions; ISO 5836:1988 Implants for surgery—Metal bone plates;
				F1622 Measuring the Torsional Properties of Metallic Bone Screws; F366 Fixation Pins and Wires; F367 Holes and Slots for Inch Cortical Bone Screws; F367M Holes and Slots with Spherical Contour for Metric Cortical Bone Screws; F382-98a Static Bending	ISO 5837-1-2 :1985 Implants for surgery—Intramedullary nailing systems; ISO 5838-1-3:1995 Implants for surgery—Skeletal pins and wires; ISO 8615:1991 Implants for surgery—Fixation devices for use in the ends of the femur in adults

Table 1.3. continued

Device	Materials of Construction: Predicate Devices and Corporate Devices/Bill of Materials	Materials Related Design Issues	Standards/Guidelines FDA	Standards/Guidelines ASTM, ANSI	Standards/Guidelines ISO
				Properties of Metallic Bone Plates; F383 Static Bend and Torsion Testing of Intramedullary Rods; F384 Static Bend Testing of Nail Plates; F897 Measuring Fretting Corrosion of Osteosynthesis Plates and Screws F1622 Measuring the Torsional Properties of Metallic Bone Screws; F366 Fixation Pins and Wires; F367 Holes and Slots for Inch Cortical Bone Screws; F367M Holes and Slots with Spherical Contour for Metric Cortical Bone Screws; F382 Static Bending Properties of Metallic Bone Plates; F383 Static Bend and Torsion Testing of Intramedullary Rods; F384 Static Bend Testing of Nail Plates; F786 Metallic Bone Plates; F787 Metallic Nail-Plate Appliances	ISO 9585:1990 Implants for surgery—Determination of bending strength and stiffness of bone plates
Biodegradable Fracture Fixation	Polylactide	Degradation rate vs. healing rate; Acid release and bone	Guidance Document for Testing Biodegradable Polymer-Fracture Fixation Devices;	F1925-98 Standard Specification for Virgin Poly(L-Lactic Acid) Resin for Surgical Implants	ISO/DIS 13781 Poly-L-lactide resins and fabricated forms for surgical implants—In-vitro degradation

Table 1.3. continued

Device	Materials of Construction: Predicate Devices and Corporate Devices/Bill of Materials	Materials Related Design Issues	Standards/Guidelines FDA	Standards/Guidelines ASTM, ANSI	Standards/Guidelines ISO
Devices	copolymers with or without biodegradable fiber reinforcement (e.g., hydroxyapatite fibers); Polyorthoesters; Polyanhydrides	resorption; particulate release; inflammation; metabolism and excretion of biodegradation byproducts	Guidance Document for testing Biodegradable Fracture Fixation Implant Devices		testing; ISO-10933 Part 9 Degradation of materials related to biological testing;
Bone Substitutes	Calcium phosphate; Hydroxyapatite and bioglass coatings and bone fillers;	Bone formation; bone adhesion; resorption/ dissolution rate of filler		F1088 Beta-Tricalcium Phosphate for Surgical Implantation; F1185 Composition of Ceramic Hydroxylapatite for Surgical Implants; F1538 Glass and Glass Ceramic Biomaterials for Implantation; F1581 Composition of Anorganic Bone for Surgical Implants; F1609 Calcium Phosphate Coatings for Implantable Materials; F1926-98 Standard Test Method for Evaluation of the Environmental Stability of Calcium Phosphate Coatings	ISO/DIS 14602 Nonactive surgical implants—Implants for osteosynthesis
Spinal Fixation Device		Stabilization of bone fracture and	Device Considerations for Spinal Fixation	F1579 Polyaryletherketone (PAEK) Resins for Surgical Implant Applications; F702	

Table 1.3. continued

Device	Materials of Construction: Predicate Devices and Corporate Devices/Bill of Materials	Materials Related Design Issues	Standards/Guidelines FDA	Standards/Guidelines ASTM, ANSI	Standards/Guidelines ISO
Systems	Stainless steels; Cobalt Chrome alloys; Titanium alloys; Carbon fiber reinforced Polysulfone or Polyetherether-keytone	bone fragments; Stress transfer; Stiffness; Resistance to bending and torsion; Fretting corrosion; Stress shielding, Bone resorption; Carbon fiber release and tissue irritation	Device Systems; Draft Guideline for Reviewing Spinal Fixation Device Systems; Draft Guideline for Reviewing Pedicle Screw Spinal Fixation Device Systems Intended for Severe Spondylolisthesis	Polysulfone Resin for Medical Applications; F1582 Spinal Implants; F1798-97 Standard Guide for Evaluating the Static and Fatigue Properties of Interconnection Mechanisms and Subassemblies Used in Spinal Arthrodesis Implants	
Dental	Stainless steels; Cobalt Chrome alloys; Titanium alloys; Nickel-based alloys; Cobalt Alloys; Gold Alloys; Calcium phosphate; Hydroxyapatite and Bioglass coatings and bone fillers; Porous coatings	Integration with bone and soft tissue; Matching bone modulus; Bone/soft-tissue/oral interface; Formation of bone vs. fibrous tissue in healing; Fracture toughness; Durability; Infection; Aveolar ridge reconstruction	Guidance Information on Surface Characteristics of Implant Metals; Guidance Information on Galvanic Corrosion of Implant Metals; Guidance to Industry and FDA Staff: Dental Cements—Premarket Notification;Guidance for Industry and FDA Staff; Dental Composites	ANSI/ADA 6-1987 (R1995) : Dental Mercury ; ANSI/ADA 69-1991 : Dental Ceramic; ANSI/ADA 5-1988 : Dental Casting Gold Alloy ; ANSI/ADA 9-1980(R1986) : Dental Silicate Cement; ANSI/ADA 33-1984(R1990) : Dental Terminology; ANSI/ADA 8-1977 (R1993) : Dental ; Dentistry—Preclinical evaluation of biocompatibility of medical devices used in dentistry—Test methods for dental materials	ISO 1559:1995 Dental materials—Alloys for dental amalgam; ISO 1560:1985 Dental mercury; ISO 1562:1993 Dental casting gold alloys; ISO 1942-2:1989 Dental vocabulary—Part 2: Dental materials; ISO 3107:1988 Dental zinc oxide/eugenol cements and zinc

Table 1.3. continued

Device	Materials of Construction: Predicate Devices and Corporate Devices/Bill of Materials	Materials Related Design Issues	Standards/Guidelines FDA	Standards/Guidelines ASTM, ANSI	Standards/Guidelines ISO
			Premarket Notification; Draft Guidance Document for the Preparation of Premarket Notification [510(k)'s] for Dental Alloys		
	2 part polymeric fillers (e.g., acrylics—chemical activation; UV activation; light activation); Zinc Polycarboxylate Cement; Glass Ionomer Cement; Zinc Silico-Phosphate Cement;	For polymeric fillers: Viscosity, heat generation, setting time, residual monomer and polymerization additives, tissue damage from heat and residuals amalgams and residual mercury; Adhesion of fillers to enamel, dentin and pulp compatibility		Zinc Phosphate Cement; ANSI/ADA 66-1989 : Dental Glass Ionomer Cements; ANSI/ADA 96-1994 : Dental Water-Based Cements; ANSI/ADA 7-1962 (R1989) : Wire Alloy, Dental Wrought Gold ; ANSI/ADA 27-1993 : Dental Materiel—Direct Filling; ANSI/ADA 41-1979 (R1989) : Biological Evaluation of Dental Materials; ANSI/ADA 57-1993 : Dental Material—Endodontic Filling Materials; ANSI/ADA 14-1982 (R1989) : Casting Alloy, Dental Chromium-Cobalt; ANSI/ADA 21-1981(R1987) : Dental Zinc Silico-Phosphate Cement; ANSI/ADA 61-1980 (R1992) : Dental	oxide/eugenol cements and zinc oxide noneugenol cements; ISO 3336:1993 Dentistry—Synthetic polymer teeth; ISO 4049:1988 Dentistry—Resin-based filling materials; ISO 6871-1:1994 Dental base metal casting alloys—Part 1: Cobalt-based alloys; ISO 6871-2:1994 Dental base metal casting alloys—Part 2: Nickel-based alloys; ISO 6872:1995 Dental ceramic; ISO 6874:1988 Dental resin-based pit and fissure sealants; ISO 6876:1986 Dental root canal sealing materials; ISO/TR 7405:1984 Biological evaluation of dental materials; ISO 7491:1985 Dental materials—Determination of colour stability of dental polymeric materials; ISO 8891:1993 Dental casting alloys with noble metal content

Table 1.3. continued

Device	Materials of Construction: Predicate Devices and Corporate Devices/Bill of Materials	Materials Related Design Issues	Standards/Guidelines FDA	Standards/Guidelines ASTM, ANSI	Standards/Guidelines ISO
	Zinc Oxide-Eugenol Cement; Mercury amalgams;			Material—Zinc Polycarboxylate Cement; ANSI/ADA 39-1992 : Dental Resin-Based Pit and Fissure Sealants; ANSI/ADA 1a-1979 (R1993) : Alloy for Dental Amalgam; ANSI/ADA 1-1977 (R1993) Alloy for Dental Amalgam; ANSI/ADA 30-1990 : Dental Zinc Oxide-Eugenol Cements and Zinc Oxide NonEugenol Cements	of 25 % up to but not including 75%; ISO 9333:1990 Dental brazing materials; ISO 9693:1991 Dental ceramic fused to metal restorative materials; ISO/DIS 9694 Dental phosphate-bonded casting investments; ISO 9917:1991 Dental water-based cements; ISO/TR 10271:1993 Dentistry—Determination of tarnish and corrosion of metals and alloys; ISO/TR 10451:1991 Dental implants—State of the art—Survey of materials; ISO 10477:1992 Dentistry—Polymer-based crown and bridge materials; ISO/TR 11175:1993 Dental implants—Guidelines for developing dental implants; ISO/DIS 11245 Dental restorations—Phosphate-bonded refractory die material; ISO/TR 11405:1994 Dental materials—Guidance on testing of adhesion to tooth structure
Periodontal Barriers			Guidance for the preparation of Premarket Notification (510K) for		

Table 1.3. continued

Device	Materials of Construction: Predicate Devices and Corporate Devices/Bill of Materials	Materials Related Design Issues	Standards/Guidelines FDA	Standards/Guidelines ASTM, ANSI	Standards/Guidelines ISO
			Resorbable Periodontal Barriers; ISO Biodegradation		
Temporo-mandibular Joint Implants			Guidance Document for the Preparation of Premarket Notification 510K for Temporomandibular Joint Implants		
Endosseous Implants			Overview of Information Necessary for Premarket Notification Submission of Endosseous Implants; 510K information needed for Metallurgical Endosseous Implants; 510K Guidance for screw type endosseous implant for prosthetic attachment		

Table 1.3. continued

Device	Materials of Construction: Predicate Devices and Corporate Devices/Bill of Materials	Materials Related Design Issues	Standards/Guidelines FDA	Standards/Guidelines ASTM, ANSI	Standards/Guidelines ISO
			Guidance for the Arrangement and Content of a Premarket Approval (PMA) Applications for an Endosseous Implant for Prosthetic Attachment		
Endosseous Implants with Bioactive Coating			Calcium Phosphate (Ca-P) Coating Draft Guidance for Preparation of FDA Submissions for Orthopedic and Dental Endosseous Implants; 510K Information Needed for Hydroxyapaptite Coated Titanium Endosseous Implants	F1185 Composition of Ceramic Hydroxyapatite for Surgical Implants; F1538 Glass and Glass Ceramic Biomaterials for Implantation	
Endosseous Implants with Porous Coating			510K Information Needed for Ti-powder Coated Titanium Endosseous Implants	F1044 Shear Testing of Porous Metal Coatings; F1147 Tension Testing of Porous Metal Coatings; F1160 Constant Stress Amplitude Fatigue Testing of Porous Metal-	

Table 1.3. continued

Device	Materials of Construction: Predicate Devices and Corporate Devices/Bill of Materials	Materials Related Design Issues	Standards/Guidelines FDA	Standards/Guidelines ASTM, ANSI	Standards/Guidelines ISO
Packaging		Microbiologic Barrier	FDA Guidelines	Coated Metallic Materials ANSI Guidelines	ISO Guidelines
Parenteral	Acrylics, Polycarbonate; PVC; Polyurethane; Polyester elastomers; Polymethylpentane; Glass				
Adhesives: Sealing Permeable Barrier to Tray	Polyolefins; Polyolefin copolymers; Acrylics; Polyurethanes				
Steam Sterilization	Tray—polycarbonate; polyester; polysulfone; Permeable barrier—				

Table 1.3. continued

Device	Materials of Construction: Predicate Devices and Corporate Devices/Bill of Materials	Materials Related Design Issues	Standards/Guidelines FDA	Standards/Guidelines ASTM, ANSI	Standards/Guidelines ISO
ETO Sterilization	nonwoven polyester; Hermetic Package—Aluminum with polyolefin layer Tray—polycarbonate; polyester; polysulfone; acrylic; PVC; Permeable barrier—nonwoven polyester				
Radiation—Gamma; E-Beam	Tray—polycarbonate; polyester; polysulfone; Permeable barrier—nonwoven polyester; Hermetic Package—Aluminum with polyolefin layer				

Central venous catheters and vascular access ports:

- Ease of infusing fluids through the device
- Puncture resistance of port septums for the totally implantable vascular access ports
- Textile/porous cuffs for tissue ingrowth and catheter stabilization
- Antimicrobial cuffs to reduce infection
- Easy repair of the externalized catheter portion for the externalized access catheters

Angioplasty catheters:

- Volume pressure relationships of balloon
- Balloon inflation times
- Balloon compliance (compliant vs. noncompliant)
- Balloon burst strength
- Guide wire drag
- Over-the-wire vs. monorail (wire through proximal third of length rather than entire catheter length) designs
- Balloon inflation of stents

These requirements will influence the design and materials required. Many times trade-offs are required to meet the most important property. Many of the balloons used are made of radiation cross-linked polyethylene or polyolefin compolymers. They are more compliant than polyester balloons, conform to the shape of the stenosis but exhibit some creep and lower burst strength than polyester balloons. Though the polyester balloons can withstand higher pressures and may be preferred for some types of calcified plaques, they have lower tear strengths and are harder to maneuver in tortuous vessels. Polyamide balloons have higher burst and tear strength than the polyolefins, but still not the burst strength of polyesters. Additional requirements of high tear strength are required for balloons utilized in stent expansion and placement.

During the design process the potential effect of unique clinical settings and diagnostic procedures on the device may need to be considered. As magnetic resonance imaging (MRI) has become more popular, including the evolving development of magnetic resonance angiography, the magnetic susceptiblity of the metallic alloys utilized in a device may need to be considered. Generally ferromagnetic and paramagnetic materials may be at risk for movement and heating in intense magnetic fields. Shellock[7] has performed an in depth review of the susceptability of medical devices.

Biomaterials and Regulatory Guidelines

Many of the regulatory guidelines will address the specific testing requirements of devices to meet both safety and efficacy. For an angioplasty catheter not only will the physical and biocompatibility issues need to be addressed, but the effectiveness of opening coronary vessels (that is "dilating" blockages) will be required in both preclinical animal studies and in controlled clinical trials. The specific regulatory requirements for angioplasty catheters are contained in the following FDA guideline: *Guidance for the Submission of Research and Marketing Applications for Interventional Cardiology Devices—PTCA Catheters, Atherectomy Catheters, Lasers, and Intravascular Stents.*

There are a variety of sources of information that relate to medical device guidelines and biomaterials that can be obtained for no or minimal cost from the Division of Small Manufacturers Assistance of the Food and Drug Administration (FDA). Information on use of the system can be obtained by calling 800 899 0381 or 301 827 0111. On-line sources of information are summarized in Table 1.4.

---

[7]Shellock FG, Morisoli S, Kanal E. MR Procedures and Biomedical Implants, Materials, and Devices, 1993 Update, Radiololgy 1993; 189, No 2:587-599.

The FDA has issued a recent guideline[8] that helps in determining when materials changes to an existing device will require a 510K. The same type of decision making will occur in deciding the need to file a PMA supplement for a class III device. As stated in the document:

...For example, a change of a material type, as discussed below, might also engender a change in the labeling of the device, e.g., the removal of a contraindication or the addition of a new warning, or a change in specifications, e.g., a reduction in the strength of the device. These collateral changes should be considered first, before applying the logic scheme described in this section. ... ...Is this a change in the type of material from which the device is manufactured? Is the generic type of material being changed? There is considerable discussion available regarding what is meant by generic materials types. FDA is developing a Biomaterials Compendium for implant devices, which will give form and structure to this discussion. The goal of this Compendium is to relate the type of device to the materials of manufacture. Appendix A[9] *to this Guidance is the latest draft of the current tables of generic materials from that Compendium and may be used by manufacturers to help in their decision-making along with this guidance. ...*

The guidance refers to ISO documents that define implant devices, ISO 10993-1, and are useful in defining biocompatibility tests. The guidance addresses material use that is supplied by specification and states:

Is the new material being supplied to a specification? If the material is being supplied to the device manufacturer's specification, a 510(k) is probably not necessary. For example, a device manufacturer might include a transparency requirement in the purchase specification for tubing to be used in an implantable catheter. Such a requirement might be related to the later processing of the tubing into the finished device. To change the supplier of that material without the need for a new 510(k), the specification should include a transparency requirement, and the device manufacturer's design validation, as required by the GMP regulation, must describe the rationale for that transparency requirement. Further, the manufacturer should document that component specifications are still met and that the performance specifications (characteristics) of the device are not adversely affected.

Also, the 510k paradigm document has been finalized[10] and provides for two faster "gateways for approval: "special 510K" and "abbreviated 510K". The "special 510K" is available if the device is a modification of a predicate device and entails submission of summaries of design control compliance. Devices that include changes in energy sources, software and dimensions are suitable for this pathway. The "abbreviated 510k" is available to devices that are amenable to device-specific guidance documents, special controls, or FDA recognized consensus standards.

The Food and Drug Modernization Act of 1997 has committed the FDA to a process of improvement and reengineering in the Center for Devices and Radiologic Health. Greater attention will be given to devices that have the most impact on public health and will utilize a risk based approach, e.g., by use of a Product Development Protocols (PDPs). The PDP will be an alternative to the PMA and allows Presubmission through the initial summary submission (Filing Review), the formal PDP submission (FDA Review), data gathering (Preclinical Phase and Clinical Phase) and to completion of the process (Notice of Completion) after which the device can be marketed (PDP completed). This process establishes an agreement between manufacturer and regulator on what preclinical and clinical testing is required prior to the marketing of a medical device.

Liability suits have impacted the supply of traditional biomaterials over the past decade. New material sources have been required, as the traditional supplies have been deleted. The

---

[8]Deciding When to Submit a 510(k) for a Change to an Existing Device; 510(k) Memorandum #K97–1; January 10, 1997

[9]Table 1.7 Biomaterials terms in proposed FDA Compendium

[10]Medical Device and Diagnostic Industry, June 1998, p. 37

qualification of alternative materials requires great expense in time and monetary resources. The process outlined in "Deciding When to Submit a 510(k) for a Change to an Existing Device; 510(k) Memorandum #K97-1; January 10, 1997", Table 1.2 and Table 1.5 can be used for identifying and qualifying new materials. The ability to match key properties to meet functional requirements of the device is of upmost importance in this approach. Materials that match chemical formulations, processing, and configurations (e.g., in yarns and textiles) will provide an easier path as an alternative material.

Some of the high publicity stories that have influenced the restriction on the uses of some materials by their suppliers have included fatigue of structural components on one type of mechanical heart valve; the use of nonbiostable polyester urethane on a breast implant; cracking of polyurethane pacemaker leads; the fragmentation of a temporal mandibular joint prosthesis fabricated with a composite fluorpolymer/carbon fiber and the controversy surrounding biological effects to silicone oil leakage from breast implants. Materials with strong restrictions on the use by particular vendors have included polyacetals, silicones, polyamides, polyester textiles and sheets, polytetrafluoroethylene and polyurethanes. Even though alternatives can be identified in some cases, device companies may need to indemnify the material suppliers. Significant resources will be needed to demonstrate that the alternative material is suitable for the design requirements of the device, including sterilization and shelf life.[11-13]

Cracking of polyurethane pacemaker leads led to vendor imposed restrictions on the sales of polyurethane for only temporary applications such as short time blood contacting catheters. Evidence emerged that many polyurethanes will undergo a slow degradation in biologic tissues, even if properly processed without exposure to excessive heat. However, harder grades of polyurethanes are more biostable. However, degradation of pacemaker insulation leads was attributed to improper extrusion conditions and enhanced by stress or the presence of metal ions released from the pacing leads which catalyzed the degradation process. A number of biostable polyurethanes have been formulated using polycarbonate soft segments rather than polyethers and are available from specialty vendors.

In breast implant recipients, adverse effects have been attributed to silicone oil leaching from silicone based breast implants. The use of silicone breast implants has become more limited since the controversy. Availability of the silicone elastomer resins from a major supplier is limited except for temporary device applications. Specialty suppliers are available.

The use of new materials without extensive implant history will require extensive testing to demonstrate long-term durability. Degradation and loss of integrity can result from hydrolysis, including enzymatic hydrolysis, particularly in the polyurethanes and polyester-based copolymers. Degradation can also occur, as discussed, by oxidation from enzymes released in wound healing and from distortion and weakening from absorption of lipids.

Polymeric materials are complex materials with ranges of molecular weights and utilizing additives to control polymerization, stability and processing. Standards developed by the International Standards Organization (ISO) have emphasized the characterization of leachables and degradation byproducts and their action on the body. The complex issues surrounding evaluation of biomaterials have been described in the literature.[14-16] The evolving issues with silicone implants is focusing on what happens to leachables including pharmacodynamics, that is where

[11]A summary of methods for shelf life studies based on materials testing can be found in: J. Donohue and S. Apostolou, "Predicting Shelf Life from Accelerated Aging Data: The D&A and variable Q_{10} Technique. Medical Device and Diagnostic Industry, June 1998; 68-72.

[12]Summary of relavent sterility guidances and validation can be found in: T. A. Ulatowski, "Device Sterility Guidances and Validation. Medical Device and Diagnostic Industry, June 1998:58.

[13]Detailed description of sterilization methodologies and medical device infections can be found in "Disinfection, Sterilization, and Preservation" Seymour Block, ed. Lippincott, Williams & Wilkins, 2000.

Table 1.4. Web sources for guidelines and standards

Regulatory Guidelines
FDA Web Page - Center For Devices: MDR's, Press Releases - http://www.fda.gov/cdrh/ 510K Home page - http://www.fda.gov/cdrh/510khome.html International Standards Organization (ISO): http://webstore.ansi.org/AnsiCatalog/AnsiCat.asp and http://www.ISO.ch/
Standards
ANSI Standards: http://www.ansi.org/ ASTM: http://www.ASTM.org FDA recognized consensus standards are listed at http://www.fda.gov/cdrh
Medical Devices
Health Industry Manufacturers Assc.: http://www.HIMANET.com Medical Device and Diagnostic Industry: http://devicelink.com/mddi
Materials Information
Society for Biomaterials: http://www.biomaterials.org/ General materials information from Drexel University: http://arvind.coe.drexel.edu/profession.html Dental information: http://www.lib.umich.edu/libhome/Dentistry.lib/Dental_tables/intro.html
Clinical Information
Cardiology including Standards of Practice: http://www.acc.org/login/index.taf American Heart Assoc.: http://www.americanheart.org/Scientific/statements/ Annals of Thoracic Surgery: http://www.sts.org/annals/toc/ Suggested Guidelines for the Practice of Arthroscopic Surgery: http:/www.arthroscopyjournal.org/guide.html General: http://www.medscape.com; http://www.theheart.org.

the leachables are going in the body, how they are changed or eliminated, and how long the process takes. Some of the biocompatibility guidelines, e.g., Tripartite and ISO, require carcinogenicity evaluation. Long term animal implants of devices required for these types of evaluation are not practical from a cost and time perspective (with at least 2 years follow-up) but may not even be realistic. In rodents and possibly larger animals, large, smooth textured implant result in tumors, a situation described as solid state tumorogenesis, which may confound the analysis. This type of tumor has not been seen in man. Screening tests for mutagenicity are available, but are not directly correlatable to tumor formation. One possible scenario for screening long term safety issues is outlined in Table 1.6. Carcinogenic potential can not be determined by this method. However, the continuing leaching of mutagenic agents over time either by the presence of a mutagenic additive or a degradation byproduct could be indicative of a possible chronic carcinogenic response.

Proposals have been set forward at various times to establish a nationwide implant retrieval system in order to help gain an understanding of how materials and devices interact in humans

Table 1.5. Biomaterials and properties

Material	Properties: Mechanical	Properties: General Properties	Applications	Issues & ASTM and ANSI Standards
Hydrogels				
Hydrocolloids	Low	Hi water content, soft, lubricious, low protein adsorption, low interfacial energy, hi vapor permeability, poor tissue adhesion	Slippery coatings for catheters, wound dressings, anti-adhesives e.g. laparoscopic applications, thromboresistant coatings, contact lenses	Fabrication - 2 part redox systems, radiation polymerization, solvent processing, sterilization, leachables, water content, lubricity, wear, durability, low molecular weight extractable oligomers, additive exractables, hypersensitivity reactions, lipid uptake, hydrolytic stability, biostability, residuals from ethylene oxide sterilization, calcification, blood element consumption, low protein adsorption, poor tissue adherence
Hydroxyethyl-methacrylate	Low			
Poly(acrylamide)	Low			
Poly(ethylene oxide)	Low			
Poly(vinlyalcohol)	Low			
Poly(vinyl-pyrrolidone)	Low			
Elastomers				
Latex rubber	Low	Elastic and extensible, hi vapor permeability, low modulus, low durometer (soft polymer), higher coefficient of friction, poly(ureaurethanes) for high fatigue resistance	Blood and urinary catheters, Intraaortic balloon pump balloons, artificial heart bladders, wound dressings, gloves, finger joints (silicones), carrier for drug delivery coatings, insulators for pacemaker leads, soft tissue implants (silicones), vascular grafts (e.g. biostable polyurethanes), heart valve components, tubing, parenteral packaging	Permanent set, creep, tacky surface, low heat stability, hysteresis on repetitive movement, tear resistance, fatigue resistance, low molecular weight extractable oligomers, additive exractables, hypersensitivity reactions (e.g. latex materials), water absorption and softening, lipid uptake, hydrolytic stability, biostability, biodegradation by-products, calcification, residuals from ethylene oxide sterilization, thermal processing, melt index, solvent processing, vulcanizing/cross-linking ASTM: F604 Silicone Elastomers Used in Medical Applications; F665 Vinyl Chloride Plastics Used in Biomedical Application; F624 Evaluation of Thermoplastic Polyurethane Solids and Solutions for Biomedical Applications
Poly(amide) elast.	Low			
Poly(ester) elast.	Low			
Poly(olefin) elast.	Low			
Poly(urethanes)	Low			
Poly(urethanes) bio-stable	Low			
Poly(vinylchloride)	Low			
Silicones	Low			
Styrene-butadiene copolymers	Low			

Table 1.5. Biomaterials and properties (continued)

Material	Properties: Mechanical	Properties: General Properties	Applications	Issues & ASTM and ANSI Standards
Plastics				
Acrylics	Mod	Low modulus, lower coefficient of friction, moderate durometer, moderate vapor permeability	Housings for extracorporeal devices (acrylics, poly(carbonates), poly(methylpentane)), catheters, angioplasty balloons, sutures, intraocular lenses, vascular grafts (polyester textiles, expanded PTFE), medical tubing, synthetic ligaments (polyester and polypropylene textiles, and ePTFE), soft and hard tissue reconstruction (acrylics, polyester and polypropylene textiles, ePTFE), membranes, (microporous poly(olefins) or PTFE) sutures, barrier packaging materials, 2 part systems for adhesives (e.g. cyanoacrylates, polyurethanes, acrylics)	Permanent set, creep, low heat stability, kink resistance of tubes, tear resistance of films (e.g. angioplasty balloons), fatigue resistance, clarity, joining/welding/solvent bonding, low molecular weight extractable oligomers, additive exractables, hydrolytic stability, biostability, biodegradation by-products, 2 part systems and cytotoxic residues, residuals from thermal processing, melt index, ethylene oxide sterilization; F639 Polyethylene Plastics for Medical Applications; F997 Polycarbonate Resin for Medical Applications; F754 Implantable Polytetrafluoroethylene (PTFE) Polymer Fabricated in Sheet, Tube, and Rod Shapes; F755 Selection of Porous Polyethylene for Use in Surgical Implants
Cyanoacrylates	Low			
Fluorocarbons	Low			
Ethylene-tetrafluoroethylene				
Ethylene-Chloro-tri-fluoroethylene				
Fluorinated ethylene propylene				
Poly(tetrafluoro-ethylene)				
Poly(vinylidene fluoride)				
Poly(amides)	Mod			
Poly(carbonates)	Mod			
Poly(esters)	Mod			
Poly(methyl pentene)	Mod			
Poly(ethylene)	Low			
Poly(propylene)	Low			
Poly(urethane)	Mod			
Poly(vinylchloride)	Low			

Table 1.5. Biomaterials and properties (continued)

Material	Properties: Mechanical	Properties: General Properties	Applications	Issues & ASTM and ANSI Standards
Engineering Plastics and Thermosets				
Epoxies	Mod	Moderate strength, high durometer (hard plastic), low vapor permeability, low creep, stiff, high heat stability for processing and heat sterilization	Structural components for bioprosthetic heart valves (poly(acetals)), acetabular cups (ultrahigh molecular weight polyethylene), bone cement (poly(methylmethacrylate)), orthopedic implants (poly(sulfone), poly(etherkeytones)), artificial heart housings; 2 part systems for adhesives (e.g. epoxies)	Fatigue resistance, creep resistance, biostability, fracture toughness, wear (e.g. acetabular cup), lubricity (e.g. acetabular cup), solvent resistance for processing, 2 part systems and cytotoxic residues, thermal processing; ATSM: F641 Implantable Epoxy Electronic Encapsulants; F702 Polysulfone Resin for Medical Applications; F1579 Polyaryletherketone (PAEK) Resins for Surgical Implant Applications
Poly(acetals)	Mod			
Poly(etherketones)	Mod			
Poly(imides)	Mod			
Poly(methylmethacrylate)	Mod			
Poly(olefin) high crystallinity	Mod			
Poly(sulfones)	Mod			
Bioresorbables				
Poly(amino acids)	Low	Hydrolytic and/or enzymatic degradation mechanisms; Hydrophobic polymers tend to degrade from surface (e.g. poly(anhydrides, poly(caprolactones), poly(hydroxybutyrates), and poly(orthoesters)	Orthopedic devices - bone plates and rods, ligaments; Sutures; Soft tissue implants for reconstructive surgery; alveolar ridge reconstuction, periodontal defect filling; Controlled drug delivery systems: e.g. growth factors for new bone formation, nanoparticles for treatment of blood vessels to prevent restenosis	Rate of bioresorption; Surface vs. bulk resorption; Particulates; Biodegradation by-products—tissue inflammation and metabolism, biodeposition and excretion of biodegradation by-products; effect of infection (acidic pH) or hematoma (basic pH) on resorption rates; Maintenance of physical properties while tissue heals. F1925-98 Standard Specification for Virgin Poly(L-Lactic Acid) Resin for Surgical Implants
Poly(anhydrides)	Mod			
Poly(caprolactones)	Mod			
Poly(lactic/glycolic) acid copolymers	Mod			
Poly(hydroxybutyrates)	Mod			
Poly(orthoesters)	Mod			
Tyrosine-derived Polycarbonates	Mod			

Table 1.5. Biomaterials and properties (continued)

Material	Properties Mechanical	General Properties	Applications	Issues & ASTM and ANSI Standards
Biologically Derived Materials				
Bovine bone	Mod	Generally thromboresistant; Xenografts generally aldehyde cross-linked but new agents (e.g. poly(epoxides), carbodiimides) under investigation; Tissue handles in fashion similar to natural tissue. Allografts generally cryopreserved; Scaffolds of decellularized allografts and xenografts can be used; Low stress state generally representative of elastin; Hi stress states of collagen	Vascular grafts, pericardial substitute; Heart valves, ligaments, tendons, bone implants; Corneal implants; Wound dressings	Biodegradation; Calcification; Immune responses if noncross-linked Allograft; improper cross-linking; or new cross-linking agent that does not block antigenic sites; Viability of cells in fresh or cryopreserved allografts; Cross-linking may stiffen material; Cytotoxic residuals from cross-linking and sterilization. Viral contamination; F1581 Composition of Anorganic Bone for Surgical Implants;
Bovine ligaments	Low			
Bovine tendon	Low			
Bovine vessels	Low			
Bovine pericardium	Low			
Decalcified human bone	Low			
Human umbilical vein	Low			
Human Bone	Mod			
Human Corneas	Low			
Human heart valves	Low			
Human skin	Low			
Porcine heart valve	Low			
Porcine skin	Low			

Table 1.5. Biomaterials and properties (continued)

Material	Properties: Mechanical	Properties: General Properties	Applications	Issues & ASTM and ANSI Standards
Bioderived Macromolecules				
Albumin	Low	Properties are a strong function of purification methods and processing; Some are processed into gels (collagen, fibrin, gelatin, hyaluronic acid) and have use for anti-adhesives. Others are used as coatings, e.g., albumin, hyaluronic acid, phospholipids) for thromboresistant coatings. Others can be processed into membranes (cuprammonium cellulose). Many are biodegradable e.g., collagen, chitosan, fibrin, gelatin.	Vascular graft coatings, utrasound contrast agent, hemodialysis membranes, experimental coatings; Lubricious coatings (e.g. Hyaluronic Acid); controlled release coatings; Wound dressings; Hybrid organs substrate, Anti-adhesives; Ocular and Joint anti-inflammatory agent, nanoparticles for intravascular drug delivery, thromboresistant coatings, sutures	Purity and inflammatory and immune responses; Biodegradation rate; Permeability of membranes; Water content of gels; Uniformity of coatings; Effect of cross-linking on inflammation, immune response, and thrombogenicity.
Cellulose acetates	Mod			
Cuprammonium cellulose	Mod			
Chitosans	Mod			
Collagen	Mod			
Fibrin	Low			
Elastin	Low			
Gelatin	Low			
Hyaluronic acid	Low			
Phospholipids	—			
Silk	Mod			

Table 1.5. Biomaterials and properties (continued)

Material	Properties: Mechanical	Properties: General Properties	Applications	Issues & ASTM and ANSI Standards
Passive Coatings				
Albumin Alkyl chains Fluorocarbons Hydrogels Silica free silicones Silicone oils		Creates biocompatible, thromboresistant coatings on polymeric and metal substrates	Thromboresistance, lubricious coatings for catheters, cannulae, needles	Adherence, wear, flaking, uniformity of coating, ability to sterilize, shelf-life, durability, shelf-life, maintaining properties in blood
Bioactive Coatings				
Anticoagulants, e.g. heparin and hirudin Antimicrobials Cell adhesion peptides Cell adhesion proteins Negative surface charge Plasma polymerized coating Thrombolytics		Creates active biocompatible, thromboresistant coatings on polymeric and metal substrates	Thromboresistance, infection resistance, enhanced cell adhesion for catheters and implants	Bioactivity, highly dependent on molecule and immobilization, biostability, adherence, wear, flaking, uniformity of coating, ability to sterilize, shelf-life, durability, shelf-life, maintaining properties in blood

Table 1.5. Biomaterials and properties (continued)

Material	Properties		Applications	Issues & ASTM and ANSI Standards
	Mechanical	General Properties		
Tissue Adhesives				
Cyanoacrylates Fibrin Molluscan glue		Chemical and physiochemical adhesion/bonding to tissue substrates; Cell adhesion sequences in fibrin and molluscan glue	Microsurgery for anastomosing vessels, vascular graft coating enhancement of cell adhesion	Viral contamination of biologic products; Filtration sterilization prior to packaging; cure time; purity and known composition (e.g. fibronectin in some fibrin glues); degree of cell adhesion and cell type; cytotoxic residuals; Degree of tissue binding
Metals and Metallic Alloys				
Cobalt chrome alloys	High	Stainless steel, cobalt chrome, nickel chrome, and titanium alloys for high strength and modulus application. Malleable alloys such as tantalum, mercurial amalgams. General corrosion resistance.	Guide wires; Mechanical heart valve housings and struts; Biologic heart valve stents; Orthopedic and dental implants and devices; Fracture plates; Nails and screws for bone repair; Vascular and urethral stents; Vena cava umbrellas; Artificial heart housings; Pacemaker leads; Leads for implantable electrical stimulators; surgical staples; Amalgams for dental fillings; Supereleastic properties of some nickel titanium formulations; Shape memory properties of some Ni titanium formulation.	Durability of passive layer; Corrosion: pitting, fretting, stress; Biocompatibility of corrosion by-products; Fracture toughness; Fatigue life; Malleability; Stiffness compared to application; Porous coatings; Nickel hypersensitivity; ASTM: F1108 Ti6Al4V Alloy Castings for Surgical Implants; F1058 Wrought Cobalt-Chromium-Nickel-Molybdenum-Iron Alloy for Surgical Implant Applications; F1295 Wrought Titanium-6 Aluminum-7 Niobium Alloy for Surgical Implant Applications; F1314 Wrought Nitrogen Strengthened-22 Chromium-12.5 Nickel-5 Manganese-2.5 Molybdenum Stainless Steel Bar and Wire for Surgical Implants; F136 Wrought Titanium 6Al-4V ELI Alloy for Surgical Implant Applications; F1377 Cobalt-Chromium-Molybdenum Powder for Coating of Orthopedic: Implants; F138 Stainless Steel Bar and Wire for Surgical Implants (Special Quality); F139 Stainless Steel Sheet and Strip for Surgical Implants (Special Quality);
Gold Alloys	High			
Mercury				
Amalgams	Low/Mod			
Nickel chrome alloys	High			
Nitinol alloys (shape memory and superelastic)	High			
Stainless steels	High			
Tantalum	High			
Titanium & titanium alloys	High			

Table 1.5. Biomaterials and properties (continued)

Material	Properties: Mechanical	Properties: General Properties	Applications	Issues & ASTM and ANSI Standards
				F1472 Wrought TI-6Al-4V Alloy for Surgical Implant Applications; F1537 Wrought Cobalt-28-Chromium-6-Molybdenum Alloy for Surgical Implants; F1586 Wrought Nitrogen Strengthened-21 Chromium-10 Nickel-3 Manganese-2.5 Molybdenum Stainless Steel Bar for Surgical Implants; F745 18 Chromium-12.5 Nickel-2.5 Molybdenum Stainless Steel for Cast and Solution-Annealed Surgical Implant Applications; F560 Unalloyed Tantalum for Surgical Implant Applications; F562 Wrought Cobalt-35 Nickel-20 Chromium-10 Molybdenum Alloy for SurgicalImplant Applications; F563 Wrought Cobalt-Nickel-Chromium- Molybdenum-Tungsten-Iron Alloy for Surgical Implant Applications; F620 Titanium 6Al-4V ELI Alloy Forgings for Surgical Implants; F621 Stainless Steel Forgings for Surgical Implants; F75 Cast Cobalt-Chromium-Molybdenum Alloy for Surgical Implant Applications; F67 Unalloyed Titanium for Surgical Implant Applications; F688 Wrought Cobalt-35 Nickel-20 Chromium-10 Molybdenum Alloy Plate, Sheet, and Foil for Surgical Implants; F961 Cobalt-Nickel-Chromium-Molybdenum Alloy Forgings for Surgical Implant Applications; F899 Stainless Steel Billet, Bar, and Wire for Surgical Instruments; F90 Wrought Cobalt-Chromium-Tungsten-Nickel Alloy for Surgical Implant Applications; F799 Cobalt-28Chromium-6Molybdenum Alloy Forgings for Surgical Implants; ANSI/ADA 6-1987 (R1995) : Dental Mercury ; ANSI/ADA 5-1988 : Dental Casting Gold Alloy ; ANSI/ADA 7-1962 (R1989) : Wire Alloy, Dental Wrought Gold ; ANSI/ADA 14-1982 (R1989) : Casting Alloy,

Table 1.5. Biomaterials and properties (continued)

Material	Properties: Mechanical	Properties: General Properties	Applications	Issues & ASTM and ANSI Standards
				Dental Chromium-Cobalt; F1813-97 Standard Specification for Wrought Titanium -12 Molybdenum -6 Zirconium -2 Iron Alloy For Surgical Implant Applications; F1341 Unalloyed Titanium Wire for Surgical Implant Applications; F1350 Stainless Steel Surgical Fixation Wire;

Table 1.5. Biomaterials and properties (continued)

Material	Properties: Mechanical	Properties: General Properties	Applications	Issues & ASTM and ANSI Standards
Ceramics, Inorganics, and Glasses				
Bioactive glasses	High	Bone bonding to many ceramic surfaces is enhanced for calcium phosphate glasses and hydroxylapatite. Bioactive glasses, tricalcium phosphates and porous hydroxylapatite are resorbable. Alumina and zirconia are inert and biostable; Electrical insulator	Bone attachment, reconstructive surgery, orthopedic and dental implants; Bone reconstruction and replacement; Carriers for bone growth factors; Alveolar ridge reconstruction; Ceramic hermetic seals for electronic packaging	Fracture toughness; fatigue life; surface lubricity for joint applications; Hi compressive strengths and generally lower tensile and bending strength; Degree of bone formation against bioactive surface and stable bioceramic surfaces; Resorption rate for bioresorbable formulations; Biostability of alumina and zirconia; ANSI/ADA 69-1991 : Dental Ceramic; F1185 Composition of Ceramic Hydroxylapatite for Surgical Implants; High-Purity Dense Aluminum Oxide for Surgical Implant Application; F1088 Beta-Tricalcium Phosphate for Surgical Implantation; F1538 Glass and Glass Ceramic Biomaterials for Implantation; F1609 Calcium Phosphate Coatings for Implantable Materials ; F1873-98 Standard Specification for High-Purity Dense Yttria Tetragonal Zirconium Oxide Polycrystal (Y-TZP) for Surgical Implant Applications;
Bioactive glass/ Ceramics	High			
Hi density alumina	High			
Hydroxylapatite	High			
Single crystal alumina	High			
Tricalcium phosphates	High			
Zirconia	High			
Carbons				
Pyrolytic (low temperature isotropic) carbon	High	Hi wear resistance, high lubricity of polished surfaces; biocompatible, thromboresistant surface; Hi strength fibers; electrical conductivity	Heart valves; Coatings; Fibers for carbon fiber reinforced plastics or carbon/carbon composites	Fracture toughness; Lubricity; Fatigue life; Wear resistance; Biostability; Low heat of protein adsorption on pyrolytic carbon
Ultra low temperature isotropic carbon	—			
Pyrolized polymers				

Table 1.5. Biomaterials and properties (continued)

Material	Properties: Mechanical	Properties: General Properties	Applications	Issues & ASTM and ANSI Standards
for carbon/carbon composites	Mod/hi			
Pyrolized fibers for fiber composites	Hi			
Composites				
Carbon fiber based:		Ability to control modulus; High strength to weight ratios; Control of anisotropic properties; Radioopaque fillers; Control of color for dental applications	Heart valve housing and struts, and stents; Housings for artificial heart; Composites to control torque and steering of catheters; Orthopedic Implants, radioopaque fillers in polymers to identify location on x-ray; Dental fillings and repair	Fiber and composite adhesion to matrix polymer; water and gas permeability; Adhesion for dental applications; Processing and joining; Fracture toughness; Fatigue life; Biostability; ANSI/ADA 9-1980(R1986) : Dental Silicate Cement; ANSI/ADA 8-1977 (R1993) : Dental Zinc Phosphate Cement; ANSI/ADA 66-1989: Dental Glass Ionomer Cements; ANSI/ADA 96-1994 : Dental Water-Based Cements; ANSI/ADA 21-1981(R1987) : Dental Zinc Silico-Phosphate Cement; ANSI/ADA 61-1980 (R1992) : Dental Material - Zinc Polycarboxylate Cement; ANSI/ADA 30-1990: Dental Zinc Oxide-Eugenol Cements and Zinc Oxide NonEugenol Cements
Epoxy	High			
Poly(ether key-tones)	High			
Poly(imide)	High			
Poly(sulfone)	High			
Radioopacifiers ($BaSO_4$, $BaCl_2$, TiO_2) blended into:				
Poly(olefins)	Low			
Poly(urethanes)	Low			
Silicones	Low			
Dental cements				
glass ionomer	Mod			
phosphates	Mod			
silicates	Mod			
zinc oxides	Mod			

Table 1.6. Overview of screening for cytotoxicity, mutagenicity, and biostability

Obtain raw materials and prepare test specimens compounded with necessary additives for fabrication, processing, and sterilization		
1) Bicompatibility testing—nonstressed samples 2) Biostability testing—stressed samples to accelerated degradation mechanisms; 37°C utilizing either physiologic buffer; serum or protein solution; calcium and/or lipid for swelling and/or calcification; or enzymes for accelerated stability testing		
In Vitro Biocompatibility Testing—Cytotoxicity; Mutagenicity; and Leachables		
	Acute in vitro < 2 days	Chronic in vitro > 1 month
Biostability testing	Acute	Chronic
	In vitro < 48 hours	In vitro > 1 month
Incoming specs Molecular weight (MW) distribution Mechanical properties (e.g., strength, elongation, tear resistance, stiffness, creep resistance,) Chemical composition	Changes in MW distribution; Mechanical properties Chemical composition	Changes in MW distribution; Mechanical properties; Chemical composition
Subcutanous Implants and Biostability Testing Samples nonstressed for Biocompatibility Samples stressed for Biostability		
—	7 day	1 month (or longer) (tumorigenic potential would require > 1yr implants, radiolabelled Polymer might be required to determine biodeposition)
MW distribution SEM evaluation for cracking Mechanical Properties Chemical Composition Leachables Histopathologic analysis		
Thromboresistance Screening		
Complement Activation In vitro platelet adhesion and aggregation In vitro flow circuits In vitro activation of coagulation Ex vitro flow circuits In vitro screening tests		

MW—Molecular weight distribution (decreasing average molecular weight would be indicative of degradation
SEM—Scanning electron microscopy

and to provide a data base of information on the biostability of materials and devices. This has also been the goal of the biomaterial compendium. The database and compendium have the potential to reduce the preclinical testing requirements of certain products. Table 1.7 lists the material terminology for the compendium. However, the variation of processing conditions and additives in polymer formulations make this a difficult task. Protection of proprietary information while making a useful database will be essential but difficult.

The issues raised by high profile complications of medical devices have resulted in a more rigorous and detailed testing program to gain approval of devices by the FDA. Certainly, rigorous testing is required when the safety of patients is concerned. However, an approach to realistic testing is required. The additional testing required will result in increased costs of development and potential lack of international competitiveness.

References

1. Helmus MN, Tweden K. Materials selection. In: Wise DL, Trantolo DJ, Altobelli DE et al, eds. Encyclopedic Handbook of Biomaterials and Bioengineering. New York: Marcel Dekker, Inc. 1995:27-59.
2. Helmus MN. Designing critical medical devices without failure. In: Spectrum, Diagnostics, Medical Equipment & Supplies, and Opthalmics. Decision Resources Inc. Nov. 6, 1992:37-1.
3. Helmus MN. Meeting demands of a leaner health care system with cost-effective medical devices. In: Spectrum, Diagnostics, Medical Equipment & Supplies. Decision Resources Inc. June 30, 1993:47-1; Futurescope III. Materials and Process Technologies; Decision Resources Inc., July 1994:III-1.
4. Helmus MN. Materials selection for medical devices. In: Spectrum, Performance Materials, Decision Resources Inc., July 5, 1993:44-1 to 44-21.
5. Helmus MN. Opportunities for biomaterials. Decision Resource Report Feb. 1995.
6. Lanza RP, Langer R, Chick WL. Principles of Tissue engineering. Austin: R.G. Landes Co. 1996.
7. Zilla P, Greisler H. Tissue engineering of Vascular Prosthetic Grafts. Austin: R.G. Landes Co. 1999.

[14]Cardiovascular Biomaterials and Biocompatibility; eds. L.A. Harker, B. D. Ratner, and P. Didisheim, Supplement, Cardiovscular Pathology, Vol. 2, No,. 3 Suppl: 53S–71S (1993).

[15]Encyclopedic Handbook of Biomaterials, Donald Wise, et al, eds., Marcel Dekker, Inc., NY, Chapter 2, 1995.

[16]Short Course, Evaluation and Testing of Cardiovascular Devices, June 12-13, 1995, M. N. Helmus Chair, A. J. Coury, Co-Chair, Society for Biomaterials, Course Notebook, 1995, Cerritos, CA.

Table 1.7. Draft controlled vocabulary from the FDA biomaterials compendium

Material Class		
metals polymers ceramics composites biological origin		
Material Subclasses		
Metals	**Polymers**	**Ceramics**
stainless steel Co & Ni allay tantalum alloy titanium alloy zirconium alloy precious/noble amalgam miscellaneous	thermoplastics thermoset/elastomers absorbable adhesive fluids	Al compound Ti compound Zr compound Ca compound carbon glass
Composites	**Biologic Origin**	
polymer matrix metal matrix ceramic matrix	tissues cells biomolecules antimicrobials	
Metals Generic Material Names		
Stainless Steels	**Co & Ni Alloys**	**Ti Alloys**
316L FeCrNiMo nitrogen strengthened ferritic martensitic austenitic	CoCrMo period CoCrWNi CoNiCrMo CoNiCrMoWFe CoCrNiMoFe	CpTi (grade 1-4) Ti 6Al 4V Ti 6Al 7Nb Ti 5Al 2.5 Fe Ti 3.8Al15Mo5Zr Nickel based Ti 13Nbl3Zr Ti 12Mo6Zr2Fe Ti 15Mo2.8Nb.2Si NiTi alloy
Zr Alloys	**Ta Alloys**	**Precious/Noble**
Zr2.5Nb	unalloyed Ta	gold silver platinum

Table 1.7. Draft controlled vocabulary from the FDA biomaterials compendium (continued)

Amalgams	Miscellaneous	
Ag-Hg	aluminum	
Cu-Sn	palladium	
	copper	
	iridium	
	mercury	
	Pt/Ir	
Polymeric Materials		
Thermoplastics	**Thermoset/Elastomer**	**Absorbable**
acetal (POM)	bis/GMA	polyester
acrylic (hydrogels)	butyl rubber	polyether
acrylic (MMA,PMMA)	epoxy	polyanhydride
fluorocarbon	EPDM rubber	polyorthoester
parylene	hydrogel based	polyetheramide
PEO hydrogel	natural latex	
poly(aryl)ether ketone	polyesterurethane	
poly(aryl)sulfone	polyetherurethane	
polyethersulfone	polyurethane (other)	
polyamide (nylon)	polyether	
polycarbonate (PC)	polyisoprene	
polyesters (PET, PBT)	polysulfide rubber	
polyester copolymer	rubber-modified acrylic	
polyethylene (PE)	silicone gel	
polyethylene (UHMWPE)	silicone elastomer	
polyimide		
polypropylene (PP)		
polystyrene (PS)		
polyurethane (PU)		
polyvinyl alcohol (PVO)		
polyvinyl chloride (PVC)		
polyvinylidine chloride		
Adhesives	**Fluids**	
acrylic based	polyvinylpyrrolidone	
cyanocrylate	silicone (PDMS)	
epoxy		
polyurethane		
silicone		
UV curable		

Table 1.7. Draft controlled vocabulary from the FDA biomaterials compendium (continued)

Ceramics and Composites Ceramics

Al Compounds	**Ti Compounds**	**Zr Compounds**	**Ca Compounds**
alumina ruby sapphire	TiN titanium carbide titanium dioxide	CaO stabilized MG-PSZ Y-TZP zirconium dioxide	Beta-TCP calcium phosphate calcium hydroxy- phosphate calcium sulfate calcium aluminate gypsum HA/TCP hydroxylapatite

Carbon	**Glass**
fibers graphite LTI pyrolytic LTI-Si alloy ULTI pyrolytic vapor deposited vitreous	bioactive glass silica based

Composites

Polymer Matrix	**Metal Matrix**	**Ceramic Matrix**
acrylic glass bis/GMA composites ceramic particle reinforced CFR epoxy CFR poly(etherketones) CFR poly(imide) CFR Poly(sulfone) CFR UHMWPE glass reinforced metal fiber reinforced PTFE composite PU/PC urethanedimethacrylate	Ag-MP35 Ta-Elgiloy wire	calcium hydroxide carbon-carbon glass ionomer cement porcelain silicate cement zinc oxide eugenol zinc phosphate polycarboxylate cement zinc

Table 1.7. Draft controlled vocabulary from the FDA biomaterials compendium (continued)

Biological Origin

Tissue	Cells	Biomolecules	Antimicrobials
blood vessel	adipocyte	agar	aminoglycoside
bone	bone marrow	albumin	antifungal
cartilage	chondrocyte	alginate	antimycobacterial
coral	endothelial	BMP	cephalosporin
cornea	epithelial	cellulose	penicillin
dura mater	fibroblast	chitosan/chitan	polymyxin
fascia lata	hepacyte	collagen	quinolone
fibrous sheath	islet	elastin	sulfonamide
heart valve	keratinocyte	fibrin	tetracycline
joint	osteoblast	fibrinogen	vancomycin
ligament/tendon	renal tubular	fibronectin	
pericardium	smooth muscle	gelatin	
umbilical cord		growth hormones	
umbilical vein		heparin	
viscera		hyaluronic acid	
		hydroxypropylmethyl cellulose	
		insulin	
		molluscan glue	
		PHB	
		phospholipids	
		polyaminoacids	
		protein extract	
		RDG protein	
		saline	
		silk	
		triglicerides, soybean oil	

CHAPTER 2

Standards and Guidelines for Biocompatibility of Medical Devices

Sharon J. Northup

Strategic management—the formulation, implementation and achievement of objectives—is essential to establishing the biocompatibility of a new medical device. The harmonization of global requirements for regulated health care products requires even more attention to regulatory strategy. This Chapter will provide an overview of the product registration requirements, standards and guidelines for biocompatibility testing, chemical characterization, and risk assessment processes that are commonly used to evaluate the safety of medical devices. It will also integrate the information derived with contemporary recommendations for assessing the potential hazards and health risks to the patient from exposure to medical devices.

The biocompatibility of medical devices has come under increasing scrutiny with the more widespread recognition that biomaterials may release substances harmful to the patient. Recent issues relating to adverse effects of the silicone gel-filled mammary implant, temporomandibular joint implants, and latex gloves have raised concerns about the sufficiency of preclinical testing. These concerns include not only the materials used to fabricate the medical device but also the durability, biocompatibility and toxicology of the materials that may be implanted for the remainder of the patient's lifetime. The magnitude of these concerns is illustrated by realizing more than 11 million Americans have an implant of some type and that implants are being placed in younger patients for longer periods of time. The use of nonimplanted medical devices is significantly higher.

Product Registration Requirements

In 1976, the U.S. Food and Drug Administration (FDA) was granted authority for the registration and regulation of medical devices. These regulations are contained in part 21 of the Code of Federal Regulations (CFR), sections 800 to 895. The strategy for registering a medical device involves identifying its human health risk classification and the appropriate process for registration. Table 2.1, which lists medical devices by medical specialty, is derived from 21 CFR sections 800 to 895. Within each medical specialty, devices are listed by the categories of general provisions, diagnostic devices, monitoring devices, prosthetic devices, surgical devices, therapeutic devices and miscellaneous devices. Class I devices are those which have limited body contact and essentially pose no significant risk. Class II devices require special controls, usually performance standards, to provide assurance of safety. A device is in Class III if there is insufficient information to determine that general or special controls are sufficient to provide reasonable assurance of its safety and effectiveness. Currently, FDA automatically places new devices that are not substantially equivalent to devices on the market prior to 1976 into Class III.

Biomaterials in the Design and Reliability of Medical Devices, edited by Michael N. Helmus

Table 2.1. Medical device classifications by U.S. food and drug administration

21 CFR Section No. Class I	Class II	Class III
862 Clinical Chemistry and Clinical Toxicology Devices b) Clinical Chemistry Test System; c) Clinical Laboratory Instruments; d) Clinical Toxicology Test Systems		
b) Alanine amino transferase (ALT/SGPT) test system, aldolase test system, delta-aminolevulinic acid, ammonia, androstenedione, androsterone, ascorbic acid, bilirubin (total and unbound) in the neonate, urinary bilirubin and its conjugates (nonquantitative), blood volume, C-peptides of proinsulin, catecholamines (total), cholesterol (total), chymotrypsin, compound S (11-deoxycortisol), copper, corticoids, corticosterone, creatinine, cystine, dehydroepiandrosterone (free and sulfate) , desoxycorticosterone, 2, 3-diphosphoglyceric acid, estradiol, estriol, estrogens, (total, in pregnancy), estrogens (total, nonpregnancy), estrone, etiocholanolone, fatty acids, follicle-stimulating hormone, formiminoglutamic acid (FIGLU), galactose, gastric acidity, gastrin, globulin, glucagon, gamma-glutamyl transpeptidase and isoenzymes , glutathione, human growth hormone, histidine, hydroxybutyric dehydrogenase 17-hydroxycorticosteriods (17-ketogenic steriods), 5-hydroxyindole acetic acid/serotonin, 17-hydroxyprogesterone, hydroxyproline, immunoreactive insulin, iron (non-heme), iron-binding capacity, isocitric dehydrogenase, ketones (nonquantitative), 17-ketosteroids, lactic acid, leucine aminopeptidase, lipase, lipid (total), lipoprotein, luteinizing hormone, lysozyme (muramidase), magnesium, malic dehydrogenase, mucopolysaccharides (non-quantitative), nitrite	b) Acid phosphatase (total or prostatic), adrenocorticotropic hormone (ACTH), albumin, aldosterone, alkaline phosphatase or isoenzymes, amylase, angiotensin I and renin, angiotensin converting enzyme (ACE), aspartate amino transferase (AST/SGOT), bilirubin (total or direct), biotinidase, blood gas (PCO2, PO2) and blood pH, calcitonin, calcium, calibrator, human chorionic gonadotropin (HCG), bicarbonate/ carbon dioxide, chloride, cholylglycine, conjugated sulfolithocholic acid (SLCG), cortisol (hydrocortisone and hydroxycorticosterone), creatine phosphokinase/creatine kinase or isoenzymes, creatinine, cyclic AMP, folic acid, galactose-1-phosphate uridyl transferase, urinary glucose (non-quantitative), glucose, urinary homocystine (non-quantitative), lactate dehydrogenase, lactate dehydrogenase isoenzymes, lecithin/sphingomyelin ratio in amniotic fluid, methylmalonic acid (non-quantitative), parathyroid hormone, phenylalanine, human placental lactogen, potassium, total protein, sodium, blood specimen collection device, thyroxine-binding globulin, thyroid stimulating hormone, free thyroxine, total thyroxine, total triiodothyronine, triiodothyronine	b) Human chorionic gonadotropin (HCG) test system (aid in the diagnosis, prognosis, and management of treatment of persons with certain tumors or carcinomas).

Table 2.1. continued

21 CFR Section No. Class I	Class II	Class III
862 Clinical Chemistry and Clinical Toxicology Devices b) Clinical Chemistry Test System; c) Clinical Laboratory Instruments; d) Clinical Toxicology Test Systems		
(nonquantitive), nitrogen (amino-nitrogen), 5'-nucleotidase, plasma mucopolysaccharides (non-quantitative), plasma oncometry, ornithine carbamyl transferase, osmolality, oxalate, urinary pH (nonquantitative), 6-phosphogluconate dehydrogenase, phosphohexose isomerase, phospholipid, phosphorus (inorganic), porphobilinogen, porphyrins, pregnanediol, pregnanetriol, pregnenolone, progesterone, prolactin (lactogen), protein (fractionation), protein-bound iodine, urinary protein or albumin (nonquantitative), pyruvate kinase, pyruvic acid, quality control material (assayed and unassayed), sorbitol dehydrogenase, testosterone, triglyceride, triose phosphate isomerase, trypsin, free tyrosine, uric acid, urinary calculi (stones), urinary urobilinogen (non-quantitative), uroporphyrin, vanilmandelic acid, vitamin A, vitamin E, and xylose test systems. c) General purpose laboratory equipment labeled or promoted for a specific medical use. Calculator/data processing module, centrifugal chemistry analyzer, continuous flow sequential multiple chemistry analyzer, discrete photometric chemistry analyzer, micro chemistry analyzer, chromatographic separation material, gas liquid chromatography system, high pressure liquid chromatography system, thin-layer chromatography system, colorimeter, photometer, or spectrophotometer,	uptake, urea nitrogen, vitamin D and vitamin B12 test systems. d) Acetaminophen, amikacin, alcohol, amphetamine, barbiturate, benzodiazepine, clinical toxicology calibrator, cocaine and cocaine metabolite, codeine, digitoxin, digoxin, diphenylhydantoin, ethosuximide, gentamicin, kanamycin, lead, lidocaine, lithium, lysergic acid diethylamide (LSD), methamphetamine, methadone, methaqualone, morphine, neuroleptic drugs radioreceptor assay, opiate, phenobarbital, phenothiazine, primiodone, propoxyphene, salicylate, cannabinoid, theophylline, tobramycin, tricyclic antidepressant drugs, and vancomycin test systems.	

Table 2.1. continued

21 CFR Section No. Class I	Class II	Class III
862 Clinical Chemistry and Clinical Toxicology Devices **b) Clinical Chemistry Test System; c) Clinical Laboratory Instruments; d) Clinical Toxicology Test Systems**		
clinical sample concentrator, beta or gamma counter, densitometer/scanner (integrating, reflectance, TLC, or radiochromatogram), electrophoresis apparatus, enzyme analyzer, flame emission photometer, fluorometer, microtitrator, nephelometer, plasma oncometer, osmometer, pipetting and diluting system, refractometer, atomic absorption, mass spectrometer, automated urinalysis system. and plasma viscometer (all for clinical use). d) antimony, carbon monoxide, cholinesterase, clinical toxicology control material, mercury, quinine, and sulfonamide test systems.		

Table 2.1. continued

21 CFR Section No. Class I	Class II	Class III
864 Hematology and Pathology Devices **b) Biological Stains; c) Cell and Tissue Culture Products; d) Pathology-Instrumentation and Accessories; e) Specimen Preparation Reagents; f) Automated and Semi-automated Hematology Devices; g) Manual Hematology Devices; h) Hematology Kits and Packages; i) Hematology Reagents; j) Products Used in Establishments that Manufacture Blood and Blood Products**		
b) Dye and chemical solution stains c) synthetic cell and tissue culture media and components, cell and tissue culture supplies and equipment, chromosome culture kit, cultured animal and human cells, mycoplasma detection media and components, animal and human sera, balanced salt solutions or formulations. d) tissue processing equipment, specimen transport and storage container, cytocentrifuge, device for sealing microsections, microscopes and accessories, automated slide stainer, automated tissue processor. e) Enzyme preparations, general purpose reagent, analyte specific reagents (unless class II or III). f) Automated blood cell diluting apparatus, microsedimentation centrifuge, automated sedimentation rate device, and automated slide spinner. g) Manual blood cell counting device, capillary blood collection tube, osmotic fragility test, and erythrocyte sedimentation rate test. h) Adenosine triphosphate release assay, leukocyte alkaline phosphatase test, leukocyte peroxidase test, thromboplastin generation test, and thromboplastin generation test. i) Blood cell diluent, lymphocyte separation medium, red cell lysing reagent, and Russell viper venom reagent.	f) Automated cell counter, automated differential cell counter, automated cell-locating device, red cell indices device, coagulation instrument, multipurpose system for in vitro coagulation studies, automated hematocrit instrument, automated hemoglobin system, automated heparin analyzer, automated platelet aggregation system, and blood volume measuring device. g) Bleeding time device, hematocrit measuring device, occult blood test, platelet adhesion test, and platelet aggregometer. h) Antithrombin III assay, red blood cell enzyme assay, activated whole blood clotting time test, euglobulin lysis time tests, factor deficiency test, erythropoietin assay, fibrin monomer paracoagulation test, fibrinogen/fibrin degradation products assay, fibrinogen determination system, erythrocytic glucose-6-phosphate dehydrogenase assay, glutathione reductase assay, hemoglobin A2 assay, abnormal hemoglobin assay, carboxyhemoglobin assay, electrophoretic hemoglobin analysis system, fetal hemoglobin assay, glycosylate hemoglobin assay, sulfhemoglobin assay, whole blood hemoglobin	f) Automated differential cell counter (for use in addition to identifying abnormal blood cells). j) Blood and plasma warming device (electromagnetic), and automated blood cell separator.

Table 2.1. continued

21 CFR Section No. Class I	Class II	Class III
864 Hematology and Pathology Devices b) Biological Stains; c) Cell and Tissue Culture Products; d) Pathology-Instrumentation and Accessories; e) Specimen Preparation Reagents; f) Automated and Semi-automated Hematology Devices; g) Manual Hematology Devices; h) Hematology Kits and Packages; i) Hematology Reagents; j) Products Used in Establishments that Manufacture Blood and Blood Products		
j) Blood bank supplies, vacuum-assisted blood collection system, blood grouping view box, blood mixing devices and blood weighing devices, cell-freezing apparatus and reagents for in vitro diagnostic use, blood bank centrifuge for in vitro diagnostic use, copper sulfate solution for specific gravity ceterminations, and heat-sealing device.	assay, heparin assay, platelet factor 4 radioimmunoassay, prothrombin consumption test, prothrombin-proconvertin test and thrombotest, prothrombin time test, sickle cell test, thrombin time test, partial thromboplastin time test. i) Bothrops atrox reagent, calibrator for cell indices, calibrator for hemoglobin or hematocrit measurement, calibrator for platelet counting, calibrator for red cell and white cell counting, and hematology quality control mixture. j) Empty container for the collection and processing of blood and blood components, processing system for frozen blood, blood group substances of nonhuman origin for in vitro diagnostic use, automated blood grouping and antibody test system, blood and plasma warming device (non-electromagnetic), automated cell-washing centrifuge for immuno-hematology, automated coombs test systems, stabilized enzyme solution, lectins and protectins, environmental chamber for storage of platelet concentrate, potentiating media for in vitro diagnostic use, quality control kit for blood banking reagents, blood storage refrigerator and blood storage freezer, and transfer set.	

Table 2.1. continued

21 CFR Section No. Class I	Class II	Class III
866 Immunology and Microbiology Devices **b) Diagnostic; c) Microbiology; d) Serological Reagents; e)Immunology Laboratory Equipment & Reagents; f) Immunological Test; g) Tumor Associated Antigen**		
c) Staphylococcal typing bacteriophage, anaerobic chamber, automated colony counter, manual colony counter, multipurpose, differential, enriched, microbiological assay, selective, and transport culture medium, automated medium dispensing and stacking device, supplement for culture media, quality control kit for culture media, microtiter diluting and dispensing device, microbiological incubator, microbial growth monitor, gas-generating device, Wood's fluorescent lamp, automated zone reader, microbiological differentiation and identification device, microbiological specimen collection and transport device. d) Acinetobacter calcoaceticus, andenovirus, arizona spp., aspergillus spp., bordetella spp., campylobacter fetus, chlamydia, citrobacter spp., citrobacter spp., corynebacterium spp., coxsackie virus, echinococcus spp., echovirus, epstein-barr virus, equine encephalomyelitis virus, erysipelothrix rhusiopathiae, escherichia coli, flavobacterium spp., influenza virus, klebsiella spp., listeria spp., lymphocytic choriomeningitis virus, mycobacterium tuberculosis immunofluorescent, mycoplasma spp., mumps virus, parainfluenza virus, poliovirus, proteus spp. (Weil-Felix), reovirus, respiratory syncytial, rhinovirus, rickettsia, rubeola (measles) virus, schistosoma spp., serratia spp., sporothrix,	b) Antimicrobial susceptibility test disc, antimicrobial susceptibility test powder, and culture medium for antimicrobial susceptibility tests. c) Coagulase plasma, and culture medium for pathogenic neisseria spp. d) Blastomyces dermatitidis, brucella spp., coccidioides immitis, cryptococcus neoformans, cytomegalovirus, entamoeba hisolytica, francisella tularensis, haemophilus spp., histoplasma capsulatum, leptospira spp., neisseria spp. direct serological test, pseudomonas spp., rabies virus immunofluorescent, Rubella virus, salmonella spp., shigella spp., streptococcus spp. exoenzyme, toxoplasma gondii, treponema pallidum nontreponemal test, treponema pallidum treponemal test, varicella-zoster virus, and vibrio cholera serological reagents. f) Albumin immunological, alpha-1-antichymotrypsin immunological, antimitochondrial antibody, antinuclear antibody, antiparietal antibody, antismooth muscle antibody, alpha-1-antitrypsin, Bence-Jones, proteins, ceruloplasmin, complement components, complement C1 inhibitor (inactivator),	c) Oxidase screening test for gonorrhea. d) Gonococcal antibody test, herpes simplex virus serological reagents.

staphylococcus aureaus, streptococcus spp., trichinella spiralis, and trypanosoma spp. serological reagents.

e) complement reagent, immunoelectrophoresis equipment, immunofluorometer equipment, immunonephelometer equipment, ouchterlony agar plate, radial immunodiffusion, rocket immunoelectrophoresis equipment, support gel.

f) Prealbumin immunological, human allotypic marker immunological, beta-globulin, breast milk, carbonic anhydrase B and C, Cohn fraction II, colostrum, factor XIII, A, S, Cohn fraction IV and V, alpha-globulin, alpha-1-glycoproteins, alpha-2-glycoproteins, beta-2-glycoprotein I, beta-2-glycoprotein III, immunoglobulin G (Fd fragment specific), lactic dehydrogenase, lactoferrin, lipoprotein X, whole human plasma or serum, plasminogen, prcthrombin, retinol-binding protein, seminal fluid (sperm), and inter-alpha trypsin inhibitor immunological test system.

complement C3b inactivator, C-reactive protein, properdin factor B, ferritin, fibrinopeptide A, free secretory component, haptoglobin, hemoglobin, hemopexin, hypersensitivity, pneumonitis, immunoglobulins A, G, M, D, and E, Immunoglobulin G (Fab fragment specific), immunoglobulin G (fc fragment specific), immunoglobulin (light chain specific), alpha-1-lipoprotein, low-density lipoprotein, alpha-2-macroglobulin, beta-2-microglobulin, infectious mononucleosis, multiple autoantibodies, myoglobin, radioallergosorbent (RAST), rheumatoid factor, systemic lupus erythematosus, total spinal fluid, thyroid autoantibody, transferrin immunological test system and tumor associated antigen.

Table 2.1. continued

21 CFR Section No. Class I	Class II	Class III
868 Anesthesiology Devices b) Diagnostic; c) Monitoring; f) Therapeutic; g) Miscellaneous		
b) Manual algesiometer, esophageal stethoscope, stethoscope head, and switching valve (ploss). f) Blow bottle, breathing tube support, nasal oxygen cannula, nasal oxygen catheter, posture chair for cardiac or pulmonary treatment, nonbreathing mask, oxygen mask, scavenging mask, Venturi mask, ether hook, gas mask head strap, breathing mouthpiece, medicinal nonventilatory nebulizer (atomizer), rebreathing device, nonpowered oxygen tent, cuff spreader, and tracheal tube cleaning brush. g) Anesthetic cabinet, table, or tray, cardiopulmonary emergency cart, nose clip, and anesthesia stool and tracheo-bronchial suction catheter.	b) Powered algesiometer, argon gas analyzer, arterial blood sampling kit, carbon dioxide gas analyzer, carbon monoxide gas analyzer, enflurane gas analyzer, gas collection vessel, halothane gas analyzer, helium gas analyzer, neon gas analyzer, nitrogen gas analyzer, nitrous oxide gas analyzer, oxygen gas analyzer, oxygen uptake computer, pressure plethysmograph, volume plethysmograph, inspiratory airway pressure meter, rhinoanemometer, diagnostic spirometer, monitoring spirometer, peak-flow meter for spirometry, gas volume calibrator, pulmonary-function data calculator, predictive pulmonary-function value calculator, diagnostic pulmonary-function interpretation calculator, esophageal stethoscope with electrical conductor, and water vapor analyzer. c) Ultrasonic air embolism monitor, Bourdon gauge flowmeter, uncompensated Thorpe tube flowmeter, compensated Thorpe tube flowmeter, gas calibration flowmeter, breathing frequency monitor, cutaneous carbon dioxide (PcCO2) monitor, nitric oxide analyzer, nitrogen dioxide analyzer, cutaneous oxygen monitor, pneumotachometer, airway pressure monitor, gas pressure gauge, gas pressure calibrator, pressure regulator, electrical peripheral nerve stimulator, differential pressure transducer, gas flow transducer,	b) Indwelling blood oxyhemoglobin concentration analyzer, indwelling blood carbon dioxide partial pressure (PCO2) analyzer, indwelling blood hydrogen ion concentration (pH) analyzer, and indwelling blood oxygen partial pressure (PO2) analyzer. c) Lung water monitor, cutaneous oxygen monitor. f) Electroanesthesia apparatus, membrane lung for longterm pulmonary support.

gas pressure transducer.

f) Emergency airway needle, oropharyngeal airway, anesthesia conduction catheter, anesthesia conduction filter, anesthesia conduction kit, anesthesia conduction needle, gas machine for anesthesia or analgesia, nitric oxide administration apparatus, laryngotracheal topical anesthesia applicator, rocking bed, anesthesia breathing circuit, breathing circuit circulator, breathing circuit bacterial filter, breathing system heater, carbon dioxide absorbent, carbon dioxide absorber, reservoir bag, breathing gas mixer, heat and moisture condenser (artificial nose), gas-scavenging apparatus, portable oxygen generator, respiratory gas humidifier, therapeutic humidifier for home use, hyperbaric chamber, flexible laryngoscope, rigid laryngoscope, anesthetic gas mask, nebulizer, esophageal obturator, portable liquid oxygen unit, powered percussor, incentive spirometer, electrically powered oxygen tent, bronchial tube, tracheal tube, tracheal/bronchial differential ventilation tube, inflatable tracheal tube cuff, tracheal tube fixation device, tube introduction forceps, tracheal tube stylet, tracheostomy tube and tube cuff, airway connector, dental protector, autotransfusion apparatus, pressure tubing and accessories, nonrebreathing valve, anesthetic vaporizer, continuous ventilator, noncontinuous ventilator (IPPB), manual emergency ventilator, powered emergency ventilator, external negative pressure ventilator, intermittent mandatory ventilation attachment, positive end expiratory pressure breathing attachment, ventilator tubing, and tee drain (water trap).

g) Portable air compressor, calibration gas, patient position support, and medical gas yoke assembly.

Table 2.1. continued

21 CFR Section No. Class I	Class II	Class III
870 Cardiovascular Devices **b) Diagnostic; c) Monitoring; d) Prosthetic; e) Surgical; f) Therapeutic**		
b) Stethoscope. d) Pacemaker service tools. e) Cardiopulmonary bypass accessory equipment, cardiovascular surgical instruments.	b) Blood pressure alarm, blood pressure computer, blood pressure cuff, noninvasive blood pressure measurement system, venous blood pressure manometer, diagnostic intravascular catheter, continuous flush catheter, electrode recording catheter or electrode recording catheter or electrode recording probe, fiberoptic oximeter catheter, flow-directed catheter, percutaneous catheter, intracavitary phonocatheter system, steerable catheter, steerable catheter control system, catheter cannula, vessel dilator for percutaneous catheterization, catheter guide wire, catheter introducer, catheter tip occluder, catheter stylet, trocar, programmable diagnostic computer, single-function, preprogrammed diagnostic computer, densitometer, angiographic injector and syringe, indicator injector, syringe actuator for an injector, external programmable pacemaker pulse generator, withdrawal-infusion pump, and thermodilution probe. c) Biopotential amplifier and signal conditioner, transducer signal amplifier and conditioner, cardiovascular blood flow-meter, extravascular blood flow probe, cardiac monitor (including cardiotachometer and rate alarm, apex cardiograph (vibrocardiograph),	b) Arrhythmia detector and alarm, catheter balloon repair kit, and trace microsphere. d) Arterial embolization device, cardiovascular intravascular filter, vascular graft prosthesis <6 mm diameter, intra-aortic balloon and control system, ventricular bypass (assist) device, external pacemaker pulse generator, implantable pacemaker pulse generator, pacemaker lead adaptor, pacemaker programmers, pacemaker repair or replacement material, annuloplasty ring, carotid sinus nerve stimulator, replacement heart valve, cardiopulmonary bypass defoamer, cardiopulmonary bypass arterial line blood filter, cardiopulmonary bypass pulsatile flow generator, cardiopulmonary bypass oxygenator, nonroller-type cardiopulmonary bypass blood pump, external cardiac compressor, external counter-pulsating device, and external transcutaneous cardiac pacemaker (noninvasive). e) Cardiopulmonary bypass defoamer, cardiopulmonary bypass arterial line blood filter, cardiopulmonary bypass oxygenator, and nonroller-type cardiopulmonary bypass blood pump. f) External cardiac compressor, external counter-pulsating device, and external transcutaneous cardiac pacemaker (noninvasive).

ballistocardiograph, echocardiograph, electrocardiograph, electrocardiograph lead switching adapter, electrocardiograph electrode, electrocardiograph surface electrode tester, phonocardiograph, vectorcardiograph, medical cathode-ray tube display, signal isolation system, line isolation monitor, portable leakage current alarm, oscillometer, oximeter, ear oximeter, impedance phlebograph, impedance plethysmograph, hydraulic, pneumatic, or photoelectric plethysmographs, medical magnetic tape recorder, paper chart recorder, apex cardiographic transducer, extravascular blood pressure transducer, heart sound transducer, catheter tip pressure transducer, ultrasonic transducer, vessel occlusion transducer, patient transducer and electrode cable (including connector), radiofrequency physiological signal transmitter and receiver, and telephone electrocardiograph transmitter and receiver.

d) Vascular clip, vena cava clip, arterial embolization device, vascular graft prosthesis of 6 mm and greater diameter, intracardiac patch or pledget made of polypropylene, polyethylene terephthalate, or polytetrafluoroethylene, pacemaker generator function analyzer, indirect pacemaker generator analyzer, pacemaker polymeric mesh bag, pacemaker charger, cardiovascular permanent or temporary pacemaker electrode, pacemaker test magnet, pacemaker electrode function tester, prosthetic heart valve holder, and prosthetic heart valve sizer.

e) Endomyocardial biopsy device, cardiopulmonary bypass bubble detector, cardiopulmonary bypass vascular catheter, cannula, or tubing, cardiopulmonary bypass heart-lung machine console, cardiovascular bypass heat exchanger, cardiopulmonary bypass temperature controller,

Table 2.1. continued

21 CFR Section No. Class I	Class II	Class III
870 Cardiovascular Devices **b) Diagnostic; c) Monitoring; d) Prosthetic; e) Surgical; f) Therapeutic**		
	cardiopulmonary bypass cardiotomy suction line blood filter, cardiopulmonary pre-bypass filter, cardiopulmonary bypass adaptor, stopcock, manifold, or fitting, cardiopulmonary bypass gas control unit, cardiopulmonary bypass coronary pressure gauge, cardiopulmonary bypass on-line blood gas monitor, cardiopulmonary bypass level sensing monitor and/or control, roller-type cardiopulmonary bypass blood pump, cardiopulmonary bypass pump speed control, cardiopulmonary bypass pump tubing, cardiopulmonary bypass blood reservoir, cardiopulmonary bypass in-line blood gas sensor, cardiopulmonary bypass cardiotomy return sucker, cardiopulmonary bypass intracardiac suction control, vascular clamp, surgical vessel dilator, intraluminal artery stripper, and external vein stripper. f) Patient care suction apparatus, embolectomy catheter, septostomy catheter, DC-defibrillator (including paddles), defibrillator tester, compressible limb sleeve, and thermal regulation system, automatic rotating tourniquet.	

Table 2.1. continued

21 CFR Section No. Class I	Class II	Class III
872 Dental Devices **b) Diagnostic; d) Prosthetic; e) Surgical; f) Therapeutic; g) Miscellaneous**		
b) Gingival fluid measurer, electrode gel for pulp testers, dental x-ray exposure alignment device, dental x-ray file holder. d) Mercury and alloy dispenser, dental amalgamator, dental amalgam capsule, preformed anchor, resin applicator, articulator, precision attachment, facebow, dental bur, dental cement, preformed clasp, preformed crown, gold or stainless steel cusp, preformed cusp, karaya and sodium borate with or without acacia denture adhesive, ethylene oxide homopolymer and/or carboxymethlycellulose sodium denture adhesive, ethylene oxide homopolymer and/or karaya denture adhesive, OTC denture cleanser, mechanical denture cleaner, OTC denture reliner, preformed gold denture tooth, resin impression tray material, dental mercury, pantograph, retentive and splinting pin, root canal post, endodontic paper point, endodontic silver point, gutta percha, posterior artificial tooth with a metal insert, and backing and facing for an artificial tooth. e) Intraoral dental drill, dental handpiece and accessories, dental diamond instrument, dental hand instrument, fiber optic dental light, dental operating light, dental injecting needle, orthodontic appliance and accessories, preformed tooth positioner, teething ring. g) Abrasive device and accessories, oral cavity abrasive polishing agent, saliva absorber, anesthetic warmer, articulation paper, base plate shellac, dental floss, heat	b) Pulp tester, caries detection device, extraoral source x-ray system, intraoral source x-ray system, cephalometer, dental x-ray position indicating device, lead-lined position indicator and sulfide detection device. d) Amalgam alloy, gold-based alloys and precious metal alloys for clinical use, resin tooth bonding agent, calcium hydroxide cavity liner, cavity varnish, dental cement (other than zinc oxide-eugenol), hydrophilic resin coating for dentures, coating material for resin fillings, OTC denture repair kit, partially fabricated denture kit, preformed plastic denture tooth, subperiosteal implant material, impression material, polytetrafluoroethylene (PTFE) vitreous carbon materials, tooth shade resin material, root canal filling resin, base metal alloy, bracket adhesive resin and tooth conditioner, denture relining, repairing or rebasing resin, pit and fissure sealant and conditioner, temporary crown and bridge resin, endodontic stabilizing splint, porcelain tooth. e) Bone cutting instrument and accessories, gas-powered jet injector, spring-powered jet injector, intraoral ligature and wire lock , bone plate, rotary scaler, ultrasonic scaler, intraosseous	d) Carboxymethylcellulose sodium and cationic polyacrylamide polymer denture adhesive, polyacrylamide polymer (modified cationic) denture adhesive, polyvinylmethylether maleic anhydride (PVM-MA) acid copolymer, and sodium carboxymethylcellulose (NACMC) denture adhesive, endosseous implant, tricalcium phosphate granules for dental bone repair, total temporomandibular joint prosthesis, root canal filling resin, glenoid fossa prosthesis, mandibular condyle prosthesis, interarticular disc prosthesis. g) Endodontic dry heat sterilizer.

Table 2.1. continued

21 CFR Section No. Class I	Class II	Class III
872 Dental Devices **b) Diagnostic; d) Prosthetic; e) Surgical; f) Therapeutic; g) Miscellaneous**		
source for bleaching teeth, oral irrigation unit, impression tube, dental operative unit and accessories, massaging pick or tip for oral hygiene, silicate protector, boiling water sterilizer, manual toothbrush, powered toothbrush, disposable fluoride tray, preformed impression tray, and intraoral dental wax.	fixation screw or wire, dental electrosurgical unit and accessories, orthodontic plastic bracket, extraoral orthodontic head-gear, teething ring (containing water). g) Ultraviolet activator for polymerization, airbrush, ultraviolet detector, porcelain powder for clinical use, cartridge syringe.	

Table 2.1. continued

21 CFR Section No. Class I	Class II	Class III
874 Ear, Nose and Throat Devices b) Diagnostic; d) Prosthetic; e) Surgical; f) Therapeutic		
b) Acoustic chamber for audiometric testing, short increment sensitivity index (SISI) adapter, earphone cushion for audiometric testing, gustometer, air or water caloric stimulator, and Toynbee diagnostic tube. d) Hearing aid, battery-powered artificial larynx, and prosthesis modification instrument for ossicular replacement surgery and nasal dilator. e) Epistaxis balloon, ear, nose, and throat burr, nasopharyngeal catheter, ear, nose, and throat manual surgical instrument, laryngostroboscope, otoscope, intranasal splint, and bone particle collector. f) Ear, nose, and throat drug administration device, ear, nose, and throat examination and treatment unit, powered nasal irrigator, external nasal splint, and antistammering device.	b) Audiometer, audiometer calibration set, auditory impedance tester, electronic noise generator for audiometric testing, electroglottograph, surgical nerve stimulator/locator. d) Hearing aid calibrator and analysis system, group hearing aid or group auditory trainer, master hearing aid, tinnitus masker, middle ear mold, partial ossicular replacement prosthesis, total ossicular replacement prosthesis, ear, nose, and throat synthetic polymer material, mandibular implant facial prosthesis, laryngeal prosthesis (Taub design), sacculotomy tack (Cody tack), endolymphatic shut, tympanostomy tube with semipermeable memberane, tympanostomy tube. e) Ear, nose, and throat: electric or pneumatic surgical drill; fiberoptic light source and carrier; microsurgical carbon dioxide laser, argon laser for otology, rhinology, and laryngology, bronchoscope (flexible or rigid) and accessories, esophagoscope (flexible or rigid) and accessories, mediastinoscope and accessories, nasopharyngoscope (flexible or rigid) and accessories.	d) Endolymphatic shunt tube with valve. f) Suction antichoke device, and Tongs antichoke device.

Table 2.1. continued

21 CFR Section No. Class I	Class II	Class III
876 Gastroenterology-Urology Devices **b) Diagnostic; c) Monitoring; d) Prosthetic; e) Surgical; f) Therapeutic**		
e) Gastroenterology-urology fiberoptic retractor, ribdam, manual gastroenterology urology surgical instrument and accessories, continent ileostomy catheter, urological clamp for males, and enema kit. f) Ostomy pouch and accessories, protective garment for incontinence, and hernia support.	b) Gastroenterology-urology biopsy instrument, stomach pH electrode, endoscope and accessories, urodynamics measurement system, gastrointestinal motility monitoring system, urine flow or volume measuring system. c) Enuresis alarm. d) Electrogastrography system. e) Fiberoptic light ureteral catheter, colostomy rod, endoscopic electrosurgical unit and accessories, gastroenterology-urology evacuator, hemorrhoidal ligator, electrohydraulic lithotriptor, mechanical lithotriptor, interlocking urethral sound, ureteral stent, water jet renal stone dislodger system, ureteral stone dislodger, urethrotome, urological table and accessories. f) Biliary catheter and accessories, suprapubic urological catheter and accessories, urological catheter and accessories, colonic irrigation system, urine collector and accessories, nonimplanted electrical continence device, esophageal dilator, rectal dilator, ureteral dilator, urethral dilator, blood access device and accessories, sorbent regenerated dialysate delivery system for hemodialysis, peritoneal dialysis system and accessories, water purification system for hemodialysis, hemodialysis system and	d) Penile inflatable implant, penile rigidity implant, testicular prosthesis. f) Implanted urinary continence device (electrical or mechanical/hydraulic), implanted blood access device, sorbent hemoperfusion system.

accessories, hemodialyzer with disposable insert (Kiil type), high permeability hemodialysis system, isolated kidney perfusion and transport system and accessories, ostomy irrigator, gastrointestinal tube and accessories and peritoneo-venus shunt.

Table 2.1. continued

21 CFR Section No. Class I	Class II	Class III
878 General and Plastic Surgery Devices **b) Diagnostic; d) Prosthetic; e) Surgical; f) Therapeutic**		
b) Speculum and accessories. d) External facial fracture fixation appliance, external prosthesis adhesive, external aesthetic restoration prosthesis, inflatable extremity splint, noninflatable extremity splint, and plastic surgery kit and accessories. e) Nonabsorbable gauze/sponge for external use, hydrophilic wound dressing, occlusive wound dressing, hydrogel wound dressing, burn dressing, surgical apparel (other than gowns and masks), introduction/drainage catheter and accessories, organ bag, surgical camera and accessories, removable skin clip, drape adhesive, eye pad, surgeon's glove, sugeon's glove cream, ultraviolet lamp for tanning, skin marker, nonpowered, single patient, portable suction apparatus, surgical microscope and accessories, surgical skin degreaser or adhesive tape solvent, removable skin staple, manual surgical instrument for general use, surgical instrument motors and accessories/attachments, suture retention device, manual operating table and accessories and manual operating chair and accessories, operating tables and accessories and operating chairs and accessories. f) Nonpneumatic tourniquets, tweezer-type epilator (electrical).	c) Surgical mesh, polytetrafluoroethylene with carbon fibers composite implant material, chin, ear, nose prosthesis, esophageal prosthesis, tracheal prosthesis. e) Surgical apparel (gowns and mask), implantable clip, cryosurgical unit and accessories, surgical drape and drape accessories, electrosurgical cutting and coagulation device and accessories, nonabsorbable gauze for internal use, absorbable poly(glycolide/L-lactide) surgical suture, surgical lamp, ultraviolet lamp for dermatologic disorders, implantable staple, powered suction pump, laser surgical instrument for use general and plastic surgery and in dermatology, absorbable surgical gut suture, nonabsorbable poly(ethylene terephthalate) surgical suture, nonabsorbable polypropylene surgical suture, nonabsorbable polyamide surgical suture, natural nonabsorbable silk surgical suture and suction lipoplasty system. f) Air-handling apparatus for a surgical operating room, needle-type epilator, pneumatic tourniquet.	d) Silicone inflatable breast prosthesis, silicone gel-filled breast prosthesis. e) Absorbable hemostatic agent and dressing, absorbable powder for lubricating a surgeon's glove, polytetrafluoroethylene injectable. f) Topical oxygen chamber for extremities.

Table 2.1. continued

21 CFR Section No. Class I	Class II	Class III
880 General Hospital and Personal Use Devices c) Monitoring; f) Therapeutic; g) Miscellaneous		
c) Bed patient monitor, stand-on patient scale, patient scale, and surgical sponge scale and Apgar timer. f) Elastic bandage, liquid bandage, hydraulic adjustable hospital bed, manual adjustable hospital bed, nonpowered flotation therapy mattress, therapeutic medical binder, burn sheet, intravascular catheter securement device, medical adhesive tape and adhesive bandage, medical absorbent fiber, neonatal eye pad, pressure infuser for an I.V. bag, non-AC-powered patient lifts, lamb feeding nipple, pediatric position holder, suction snakebite kit, medical support stocking, therapeutic scrotal support, umbilical occlusion device and lice removal kit. g) Absorbent tipped applicator, ice bag, medical disposable bedding, bed board, cardiopulmonary resuscitation board, hot/cold water bottle, medical chair and table, ultrasonic cleaner for medical instruments, cast cover, mattress cover for medical purposes, ring cutter, tongue depressor, patient examination glove, examination gown, medical insole, patient lubricant, skin pressure protectors, body waste receptacle, protective restraint, manual patient transfer device, washers for body waste receptacles, medical disposable scissors, hand-carried stretcher, irrigating syringe, liquid crystal vein locator, vein stabilizer and infusion stand.	c) Liquid crystal forehead temperature stip, electronic monitor for gravity flow infusion systems, electrically powered spinal fluid pressure monitor, spinal fluid manometer, sterilization process indicator, clinical color change thermometer, clinical electronic thermometer, clinical mercury thermometer. f) I.V. container, medical recirculating air cleaner, AC-powered adjustable hospital bed, pediatric hospital bed, infant radiant warmer, intravascular catheter, neonatal incubator, neonatal transport incubator, nonelectrically powered fluid injector, intravascular administration set, patient care reverse isolation chamber, jet lavage, AC-powered patient lift, alternating pressure air flotation mattress, temperature regulated water mattress, hypodermic single lumen needle, acupuncture needle, neonatal phototherapy unit, infusion pump, medical support stocking, piston syringe. g) Ethylene oxide gas aerator cabinet, AC-powered medical examination light, medical ultraviolet air purifier, medical ultraviolet water purifier, vacuum-powered body fluid suction apparatus, powered patient transfer device, sterilization wrap, ethylene oxide gas sterilizer, dry-heat sterilizer, steam sterilizer, wheeled stretcher, syringe needle introducer.	f) Chemical cold pack, and snakebite kit.

Table 2.1. continued

21 CFR Section No. Class I	Class II	Class III
882 Neurological Devices b) Diagnostic; e) Surgical; f) Therapeutic		
b) Ataxiagraph, two-point discriminator, electroencephalogram (EEG) signal spectrum analyzer, electroencephalograph test signal generator, esthesiometer, tuning fork, percussor, pinwheel, and ultrasonic scanner calibration test block. e) Skull plate anvil, ventricular cannula, neurosurgical chair, clip forming/cutting instrument, clip removal instrument, clip rack, neurosurgical headrests, cranioplasty material forming instrument, microsurgical instrument, nonpowered neurosurgical instrument, shunt system implantation instrument, leukotome, neurosurgical suture needle, skull punch, and skull plate screwdriver.	b) Rigidity analyzer, echoencephalograph, electroconductive media, cortical, cutaneous, depth, nasopharyngeal, and needle electrode, electroencephalograph, electroencephalograph electrode/lead tester, nystagmograph, neurological endoscope, galvanic skin response measurement device, nerve conduction velocity measurement device, skin potential measurement device, powered direct-contact temperature measurement device, alpha monitor, intracranial pressure monitoring device, physiological signal amplifier, physiological signal conditioner, evoked response electrical, mechanical, photic stimulator and auditory stimulator, tremor transducer and electroencephalogram (EEG) telemetry system. c) Ventricular catheter, scalp clip, aneurysm clip applier, cryogenic surgical device, dowel cutting instrument, manual cranial drills, burrs, trephines, and their accessories, powered compound cranial drills, burrs, trephines, and their accessories, powered simple cranial drills, burrs, trephines and their accessories, cranial drill handpiece (brace), electric or pneumatic cranial drill motor, radiofrequency lesion generator, neurosurgical head holder (skull clamp), stereotaxic instrument, cottonoid paddie, radiofrequency lesion probe,	b) Ocular plethysmograph, rheoencephalograph f) Intravascular occluding catheter, cranial electrotherapy stimulator, implanted cerebellar stimulator, implanted diaphragmatic/phrenic nerve stimulator, implanted intracerebral/ subcortical stimulator for pain relief, implanted spinal cord stimulator for bladder evacuation, implanted neuromuscular stimulator, implanted spinal cord stimulator for pain relief, electroconvulsive therapy device, and artificial embolization device.

Table 2.1. continued

21 CFR Section No. Class I	Class II	Class III
882 Neurological Devices **b) Diagnostic; e) Surgical; f) Therapeutic**		
	self-retaining retractor for neurosurgery, manual and powered rongeur. f) Methyl methacrylate for aneurysmorrhaphy, biofeedback device, bite block, carotid artery clamp, aneurysm and implanted malleable clip, aversive conditioning device, burr hole cover, nerve cuff, methyl methacrylate for cranioplasty, preformed alterable or nonalterable cranioplasty plate, cranioplasty plate fastener, lesion temperature monitor, central nervous system fluid shunt and components, external functional neuromuscular stimulator, implanted peripheral, spinal cord, and transcutaneous electrical nerve stimulator for pain relief. Preformed craniosynostosis strip, dura substitute, skull tongs for traction and cranial orthosis.	

Table 2.1. continued

21 CFR Section No. Class I	Class II	Class III
884 Obstetrical and Gynecological Devices **b) Diagnostic; c) Monitoring; d) Prosthetic; e) Surgical; f) Therapeutic; g) Assisted reproductive devices**		
b) Viscometer for cervical mucus. c) Fetal stethoscope, telethermographic system, and liquid crystal thermographic system. e) Obstetric-gynecologic general manual instrument. f) Nonpowered breast pump, unscented menstrual pad, and vaginal insufflator. g) Assisted reproductive microscopes and microscope accessories.	b) Endometrial aspirator, endometrial brush, endometrial washer, endocervical aspirator, endometrial suction curette and accessories, uterotubal carbon dioxide insufflator and accessories, perineometer, amniotic fluid sampler (amniocentesis tray), fetal blood sampler, colposcope, culkoscope and accessories, transcervical endoscope (amnioscope) and accessories, hysteroscope and accessories, hysteroscopic insufflator, gynecologic laparoscope and accessories, laparoscopic insufflator. c) Obstetric-gynecologic ultrasonic imager, fetal cardiac monitor, fetal phonocardiographic monitor and accessories, fetal ultrasonic monitor and accessories, fetal scalp circular (spiral) electrode and applicator, intrauterine pressure monitor and accessories, external uterine contraction monitor and accessories, perinatal monitoring system and accessories, obstetric ultrasonic transducer and accessories. d) Cervical drain, vaginal pessary, fallopian tube prosthesis, vaginal stent. e) Gynecologic electrocautery and accessories, unipolar endoscopic coagulator-cutter and accessories, hygroscopic laminaria cervical dilator, fetal vacuum extractor, obstetric forceps,	b) Transabdominal amnioscope (fetoscope) and accessories. c) Obstetric data analyzer, fetal electroencephalogram monitor, fetal scalp clip electrode and applicator. e) Expandable cervical dilator, vibratory cervical dilators. f) Abdominal decompression chamber, glans sheath, contraceptive intrauterine device (IUD) and introducer, contraceptive tubal occlusion device (TOD) and introducer, powered vaginal muscle stimulator.

obstetric fetal destructive instrument, obstetric-gynecologic specialized manual instrument, gynecologic surgical laser, obstetric table and accessories, endoscopic electrocautery and accessories, bipolar endoscopic coagulator-cutter and accessories.

f) Vacuum abortion system, obstetric anesthesia set, powered breast pump, cervical cap, condom, condom with spermicidal lubricant, contraceptive diaphragm and accessories, perineal heater, menstrual cup, scented or scented deodorized menstrual pad, scented or scented deodorized menstrual tampon, unscented menstrual tampon, therapeutic vaginal douche apparatus, genital vibrator for therapeutic use.

g) Assisted reproduction needles, catheters, accessories, microtools, micropipette fabrication instruments, micromanipulators and microinjectors, labware, water and water purification systems, reproductive media and supplements.

Table 2.1. continued

21 CFR Section No. Class I	Class II	Class III
886 Ophthalmic Devices b) Diagnostic; d) Prosthetic; e) Surgical; f) Therapeutic		
b) Ocular esthesiometer, adaptometer (biophotometer), anomaloscope, Haidlinger brush, ophthalmic chair, visual acuity chart, color vision plate illuminator, color vision tester, distometer, optokinetic drum, euthyscope (battery powered), exophthalmometer, fixation device, fornixscope, Amsler grid, haploscope, keratoscope, Bagolini lens, diagnostic condensing lens, flexible diagnostic Fresnel lens, diagnostic Hruby fundus lens, Maddox lens, ophthalmic trial lens set, ophthalmic trail lens clip, ophthalmic trail lens frame, ophthalmic lens gauge, lens measuring instrument, ophthalmic contact lens radius measuring device, Maxwell spot, corneal radius measuring device, stereopsis measuring instrument, headband mirror, perimeter, ophthalmic bar prism, ophthalmic Fresnel prism, gonioscopic prism, ophthalmic rotary prism, ophthalmic projector, pupillograph, pupillometer, ophthalmic refractometer, manual refractor, retinoscope, nearpoint ruler, Schirmer strip, tangent screen (campimeter), stimulatan (including crossed cylinder), ophthalmic instrument stand, stereoscope, fusion and stereoscopy target, nystagmus tape, spectacle dissociation test system, tonometer sterilizer, and transilluminator. e) Powered corneal burr, ophthalmic knife test drum, ophthalmic electrolysis unit, intraocular lens guide, operating headlamp, manual ophthalmic surgical	b) Corneal electrode, euthyscope (AC powered), afterimage flasher, visual field laser instrument, polymethylmethacrylate (PMMA) diagnostic contact lens, eye movement monitor, ophthalmoscope, AC-powered photostimulator, ophthalmic preamplifier, ophthalmic isotope uptake probe, skiascopic rack, AC powered slitlamp biomicroscope, tonometer and accessories, transilluminator. d) Ophthalmic tantalum clip, ophthalmic conformer, artificial eye, absorbable implant (scleral buckling method), eye sphere implant, extraocular orbital implant, keratoprosthesis, aqueous shunt and scleral shell. e) Radiofrequency electrosurgical cautery apparatus, thermal cautery unit, vitreous aspiration and cutting instrument, cryophthalmic unit, ophthalmic electrolysis unit, operating headlamp, ophthalmic laser, Nd:YAG laser for posterior capsulotomy, electronic metal locator, AC-powered magnet, ocular pressure applicator, phacofragmentation system, ophthalmic photocoagulator, ophthalmic sponge, ophthalmic beta radiation source.	d) Intraocular lens, eye valve implant. e) Intraocular gas, intraocular fluid, intraocular pressure measuring device. f) Contact lenses for extended wear.

instrument, ocular surgery irrigation device, keratome, permanent magnet, ophthalmic surgical marker, ophthalmic eye shield, ophthalmic operating spectacles, and ophthalmic instrument table. f) Low-power binocular loupe, contact lens inserter/remover, low-vision magnifier, ptosis crutch, ophthalmic bar reader, ophthalmic prism reader, closed-circuit television reading system, magnifying spectacles, spectacle frame, prescription spectacle lens, sunglasses (nonprescription), low-vision telescope, electronic vision aid, image intensification vision, and optical vision aid.	f) Rigid gas permeable contact lens, soft (hydrophilic) contact lens (daily wear), soft (hydrophilic) contact lens care products.

Table 2.1. continued

21 CFR Section No. Class I	Class II	Class III
888 Orthopedic Devices b) Diagnostic; d) Prosthetic; e) Surgical		
b) Nonpowered dynamometer, and goniometer. e) Calipers for clinical use, cement dispenser, cement mixer, cement monomer vapor evacuator, cement ventilation tube, depth gauge for clinical use, orthopedic manual surgical instrument, protractor for clinical use, template for clinical use, nonpowered orthopedic traction apparatus and accessories, noninvasive traction component, cast component, cast removal instrument, manual cast application and removal instrument.	b) Arthroscope, AC-powered dynamometer. d) Bone cap, bone fixation cerclage, bone heterograft, intramedullary fixation rod, passive tendon prosthesis, single/multiple component metallic bone fixation appliances and accessories, smooth or threaded metallic bone fixation fastener, spinal interlaminal fixation orthosis, spinal intervertebral body fixation orthosis, pedicle screw spinal system, ankle joint metal/composite semi-constrained cemented prosthesis, ankle joint metal/polymer semi-constrained cemented prosthesis, elbow joint metal/polymer semi-constrained cemented prosthesis, finger joint polymer constrained prosthesis, hip joint metal/composite semi-constrained cemented prosthesis, hip joint metal/ceramic/polymer semi-constrained cemented or nonporous uncemented prosthesis, hip joint femoral (hemi-hip) metallic cemented or uncemented prosthesis, hip joint femoral (hemi-hip) cemented or uncemented prosthesis, hip joint femoral (hemi-hip) metallic resurfacing prosthesis, hip joint metal/polymer semi-constrained cemented prosthesis, hip joint metal/polymer/metal semi-constrained porous-coated uncemented prosthesis, hip joint metal/polymer semi-constrained resurfacing cemented prosthesis,	d) Bone heterograft, polymethylmethacrylate (PMMA) bone cement. Ankle joint metal/polymer non-constrained cemented prosthesis. Elbow metal/metal or metal polymer constrained cemented prosthesis. Elbow joint humeral (hemi-elbow) metallic uncemented prosthesis. Finger joint metal/metal constrained uncemented prosthesis. Finger joint metal/metal constrained cemented prosthesis. Hip joint metal constrained cemented or uncemented prosthesis. Hip joint metal/polymer constrained cemented or uncemented prosthesis. Hip joint metal/metal semi-constrained, with a cemented acetabular component, prosthesis. Hip joint metal/metal semi-constrained, with an uncemented acetabular component, prosthesis. Hip joint femoral (hemi-hip) trunnion-bearing metal/polyacetal cemented prosthesis. Knee joint femorotibial metallic constrained cemented prosthesis. Knee joint femoral/hemi-knee, metallic uncemented prosthesis. Shoulder joint metal/metal or metal/polymer constrained cemented prosthesis. Shoulder joint glenoid (hemi-shoulder) metallic cemented prosthesis.

knee joint femorotibial metal/composite non-constrained cemented prosthesis, knee joint femorotibial metal/composite semi-constrained cemented prosthesis, knee joint femorotibial metal/polymer constrained cemented prosthesis, knee joint femorotibial metal/polymer non-constrained cemented prosthesis, knee joint femorotibial metal/polymer non-constrained cemented prosthesis, knee joint femorotibial metal/polymer semi-constrained cemented prosthesis, knee joint patellofemoral polymer/metal semi-constrained cemented prosthesis, knee joint patellofemorotibial polymer/metal/polymer semi-constrained cemented prosthesis, knee joint tibial (hemi-knee) metallic resurfacing uncemented prosthesis, knee joint patello-femorotibial polymer/metal constrained cemented prosthesis, knee joint patellar (hemi-knee) metallic resurfacing uncemented prosthesis, shoulder joint humeral (hemi-shoulder) metallic uncemented prosthesis, toe joint polymer constrained prosthesis, shoulder joint metal/polymer non-constrained cemented prosthesis, shoulder joint metal/polymer semi-constrained cemented prosthesis, toe joint phalangeal (hemi-toe) polymer prosthesis, wrist joint carpal lunate and scaphoid polymer prosthesis, wrist joint carpal trapezium polymer prosthesis, wrist joint polymer constrained prosthesis, wrist joint metal constrained cemented prosthesis, wrist joint metal/polymer semi-constrained cemented prosthesis, wrist joint ulnar (hemi-wrist polymer prosthesis).

e) sonic surgical instrument and accessories/attachments.

Table 2.1. continued

21 CFR Section No. Class I	Class II	Class III
890 Physical Medicine Devices b) Diagnostic; d) Prosthetic; f) Therapeutic		
b) Electrode cable. d) Prosthetic and orthotic accessory, cane, mechanical chair, crutch, flotation cushion, external limb orthotic component, external limb prosthetic component, limb orthosis, truncal orthosis, plinth, arm sling, congenital hip dislocation abduction splint, Denis Brown splint, nonpowered communication system, mechanical table, cane, crutch, walker tips and pads, mechanical walker, and mechanical wheelchair, wheelchair accessory, wheelchair component, wheelchair platform scale. f) Daily activity assist device, nonpowered sitz bath, manual patient rotation, exercise component, nonmeasuring exercise equipment, cold pack, hot or cold disposable pack, moist heat pack, pressure-applying device, and traction accessory.	b) Chronaximeter, diagnostic electromyograph, diagnostic electromyograph needle electrode, powered reflex hammer, force-measuring platform, intermittent pressure measurement system, miniature pressure transducer, diagnostic muscle stimulator, isokinetic testing and evaluation system. d) Electric positioning chair, external assembled lower limb prosthesis, powered wheeled stretcher, powered communication system, powered environmental control system, powered table, motorized three-wheeled vehicle, powered wheelchair, special grade wheelchair, standup wheelchair, wheelchair elevator. f) Immersion hydrobath, paraffin bath, powered patient transport, air-fluidized bed, powered flotation therapy bed, powered patient rotation bed, moist steam cabinet, microwave diathermy, shortwave diathermy, ultrasonic diathermy, measuring exercise equipment, powered exercise equipment, powered finger exerciser, infrared lamp, iontophoresis device, powered external limb overload warning device, powered inflatable tube massager, therapeutic massager, water circulating hot or cold pack, powered heating pad, powered muscle stimulator, ultrasound and muscle stimulator, multi-function physical therapy table, power traction equipment, chilling unit, powered	d) Rigid pneumatic structure orthosis, stair-climbing wheelchair.

Table 2.1. continued

21 CFR Section No. Class I	Class II	Class III
892 Radiology Devices **b) Diagnostic; f) Therapeutic; g) Miscellaneous**		
b) Scintillation (gamma) camera, positron camera, nuclear whole body counter, nuclear rectilinear scanner, nuclear uptake probe, nuclear whole body scanner, nuclear scanning bed, nuclear anthropomorphic phantom, nuclear flood source phantom, nuclear sealed calibration source, nuclear electrocardiograph synchronizer, radionuclide test patter phantom, radiographic film marking system, radiographic film, radiographic film illuminator, radiographic grid, radiographic head holder, medical image storage device, medical image communications device, radiologic quality assurance instrument, radiographic anthropomorphic phantom, radiographic intensifying screen, and radiographic ECG/respirator synchronizer, radiologic table. f) Manual radionuclide applicator system, and radionuclide teletherapy source. g) Personnel protective shield.	heating unit, therapeutic vibrator. b) Magnetic resonance diagnostic device, bone densitometer, emission computed tomography system, fluorescent scanner, nuclear tomography system, radionuclide dose calibrator, radionuclide rebreathing system, nonfetal ultrasonic monitor, ultrasonic pulsed doppler imaging system, ultrasonic pulsed echo imaging system, diagnostic ultrasonic transducer, angiographic x-ray system, diagnostic x-ray beam-limiting device, cine or spot fluorographic x-ray camera, image-intensified fluoroscopic x-ray system, non-image intensified fluoroscopic x-ray system, spot-film device, stationary x-ray system, diagnostic x-ray high voltage generator, mammographic x-ray system, mobile x-ray system, photofluorographic x-ray system, tomographic x-ray system, computed tomography x-ray system, diagnostic x-ray tube housing assembly, diagnostic x-ray tube mount, pneumoencephalographic chair, radiologic patient cradle, radiographic film cassette, radiographic film/cassette changer, radiographic film/cassette changer programmer, wall-mounted radiographic cassette holder, automatic radiographic file processor, transilluminator for breast evaluation, medical image digitizer, medical image hard copy device, picture archiving and communications service. f) Medical charged-particle radiation therapy	

Table 2.1. continued

21 CFR Section No. Class I	Class II	Class III
892 Radiology Devices b) Diagnostic; f) Therapeutic; g) Miscellaneous		
	system, medical neutron radiation therapy system, remote controlled radionuclide applicator system, radiation therapy beamshaping block, radionuclide brachytherapy source, radionuclide radiation therapy system, powered radiation therapy patient support assembly, light beam patient position indicator, radiation therapy simulation system, x-ray radiation therapy system, therapeutic x-ray tube housing assembly.	

Source: http://www.access.gov.gpo.gov/nara/cfr
Accessed February 2001.

The major processes for a commercial organization to submit information about a medical device to the FDA are preamendment device listing, 510(k) premarket notification, investigational device exemptions (IDE), and premarket approval (PMA) applications. The listing of preamendment devices, which occurred in the years immediately following the enactment of the legislation, required the applicant to provide evidence that the firm marketed the device prior to 1976. This evidence included design specifications, manufacturing processes, marketing materials, catalogs, and sales or shipping documents. The 510(k), IDE, or PMA submissions are used for devices placed in commerce by any other manufacturer after 1976. The 510(k) notification from a new manufacturer must supply biocompatibility information on the device or certification that the materials are substantially equivalent to the legally marketed device and are identically processed or sterilized as well as other requirements. The applicant may substitute technologically improved materials in 510(k) classified preamendment devices with supporting documentation instead of simply duplicating marketed products. PMA applications typically require clinical trials in humans along with biocompatibility testing of the medical device. The principal distinction between the role of the 510(k) notification and the PMA application is that if substantial equivalence is demonstrated, then the device is assumed to be safe and effective. If substantial equivalence cannot be demonstrated, then the FDA will require a PMA application, which contains reasonable evidence to support a determination of safety and effectiveness.

There are many fine points to the registration and classification of a medical device. The application for approval of medical devices is generally submitted to the FDA Center for Device and Radiological Health (CDRH). However, if the device is utilized in or indicated for the collection, processing or administration of biological products (e.g., blood or blood components), then the application is reviewed by FDA's Center for Biologics Evaluation and Research (CBER). Devices that are used in combination with a drug product are subjected to review by both CDRH and FDA's Center for Drug Evaluation and Research (CDER). For example, the extracorporeal device for ultraviolet irradiation of a patient's own white blood cells during treatment of psoriasis was registered as a drug therapy with CDER rather than a Class III medical device (Freiherr, 1997). That is, the drug product for the therapy, i.e., 8-methoxypsoralen, was registered and the dossier included a premarket application for the ultraviolet irradiation device including design specifications, performance characteristics, safety, and effectiveness. Similar devices for ultraviolet or gamma irradiation of blood components that are transfused into a patient other than the donor are classified as medical devices and are reviewed by CDRH with consultation of experts in CBER. Intercenter agreements among the three FDA centers are available to assist in identifying the lead division when it is likely that the medical devices will be of interest to more than one center. The interested reader is encouraged to consult the FDA Division of Small Manufacturers Assistance (DSMA) for specific information including guidance documents for specific devices, detailed requirements for submitting applications, intercenter agreements, compliance issues, proposals for new guidance documents, or regulations published in the U.S. Federal Register. Despite the name, DSMA is the front door for all companies for submission-specific questions, general information on basic issues, and documents. The division may be accessed at the Internet address of http://www.fda.gov.

Certification that a medical device contains a biomaterial that has been used in other FDA cleared products for quite some time can possibly avoid submission of detailed biocompatibility testing. However, there is a risk involved in claiming that the biomaterials in the device submitted for 510(k) notification are identically processed or sterilized without detailed information concerning a predicate device's biomaterials. Some of the conditions that should be met are that the risk of a device is low, the material is well-recognized with a long history of use, the manufacturing process does not introduce any toxic contaminants into the material to the best of the applicant's knowledge, or there is information in the firm's files demonstrating a good faith basis for the statements made in the certification that the materials, and material-processing techniques are identical to those of the predicate device. If the vendor of the materials has a device master file on record with the FDA, it is also acceptable for the applicant to provide a letter from the vendor permitting FDA to access the master file. When the certification or device master file requirements cannot be met, the manufacturer must provide preclinical biocompatibility testing information on the medical device.

Standards and Guidelines for Biocompatibility Testing

The requirements for biocompatibility testing have been harmonized internationally under the aegis of the International Organization for Standardization (ISO). Participants in the working groups represented all of the developed nations and many developing nations. The master list of recommendations is contained in ISO 10993-1 Biological evaluation of Medical Devices-Part 1: Evaluation and testing. This standard lists a series of biological assays to be performed by the manufacturer to demonstrate a particular device is safe for its intended use. Parts 2 through 18 of ISO 10993 contain guidelines on the conduct of the assays (Table 2.2). In some cases, parts 2 through 18 are specific and prescriptive whereas others provide general directions and cross-reference more specific standards. The latter situation occurs whenever the topic is very complex and there are a variety of detailed, extant standards available for reference.

Individual countries subsequently adopted the harmonized requirements or modified the standards to mesh with the regulatory infrastructure and philosophy of that nation or economic community (i.e., national standards). The European Community retained many of the standards as harmonized. Japan adopted ISO 10993-1 as published but made major changes in the conduct of the individual biological assays (see Chapter 4). The U.S. regulatory requirements for biocompatibility testing are published in FDA's Blue Book Memorandum #G95-1, dated May 1, 1995. Key differences are FDA's requirement for in vivo testing for selected device categories (i.e., systemic toxicity, subchronic toxicity, implantation, material-mediated pyrogenicity in vivo, and genotoxicity; see Tables 2.3 and 2.4). Specific examples of differences between the FDA and ISO guidelines include surface devices permanently contacting mucosal membranes (e.g., intrauterine devices) and devices with prolonged or permanent contact with tissue/bone/dentin (e.g., dental cements and filling materials).

The matrices in the FDA and ISO documents are to be considered on a case-by-case basis and are not proscriptive. The basic requirement in the guidelines is that selected bioassays "shall be considered." If a specified assay is not performed, then the requirement is a document to explain why the assay was not performed. That is, not all of the tests suggested in the matrices are essential and relevant for all devices and, moreover, the tests suggested may not be sufficient for a specific medical device. The FDA, ISO and Japanese documents set forth seven fundamental principles for the evaluation of medical devices and provide a framework for their application (see Table 2.5). Medical devices are classified based upon three factors: the nature of the device's contact with the body (i.e., surface, externally communicating, or internal contact); the duration of the device-body contact (i.e., transient, short-term or long-term); and the type of materials used in the device (e.g., polymers). The more invasive the route of exposure or the more extensive the duration of use, the greater the number of biological tests and the longer their duration. The design of biocompatibility and toxicity studies to support a device application can be crucial to timely approval. These studies should use the appropriate species and an appropriate number of animals to demonstrate biocompatibility and the lack of toxicity. The testing should include negative controls and either positive controls or a reference device that has been in commerce and shown to have no adverse clinical effects, where appropriate. These controls may aid in determining whether the outcomes of the biocompatibility testing are related to the test procedure or the medical device or biomaterial. All studies, including preliminary and exploratory investigations, should be done with an understanding that the data may be subjected to regulatory review. It is desirable that all toxicology studies comply with FDA's Good Laboratory Practice (GLP) regulation (21 CFR part 58) and/or the Organization for Economic Cooperation and Development GLP standard for international submissions. The data should be subjected to appropriate biostatistical analyses and contain sufficient detail to permit a reviewer to confirm the statistical analyses. FDA's guidance document, "Observed uses and abuses of statistical procedures in medical device submissions" and the GLP regulations both emphasize the need for appropriate biostatistical analyses.

For specific medical devices, individual product standards (also known as vertical standards), guidance documents, or toxicology profiles may be available from the FDA, ISO, American Society of Testing and Materials (ASTM), American Association for the Advancement of Medical Instrumentation (AAMI) and other national standards development organizations in Europe, Japan, or other countries. The guidance documents of individual device classes may have more exacting requirements than the requirements in the biocompatibility standards. For example, the FDA's guidance on hemodialyzers requires "Consideration...[of]...the possibility of the release of toxic substances and particulate that might accumulate during the manufacturing, sterilization and/or reprocessing processes. Materials in contact with either the blood or the dialysate should be tested for leachability and toxicity, and evaluated for mutagenicity, carcinogenicity, and immune sensitization, as relevant. All leachables should be identified, and whenever possible, quantified..." (FDA, 1994). Similarly, the FDA's guidance document on vascular grafts contains device specific requirements beyond those of the biocompatibility documents (FDA, 1993). That is, the guidance requires biocompatibility and toxicological characterization of sterilization and residual chemicals used in the manufacture of the graft and any biodegradation byproducts formed after implantation. The concerns for the ultimate fate, quantities, sites/organs of deposition, routes of excretion, and potential clinical significance of polymer, biodegradation byproducts, and metabolites also emphasize the need for histopathological evaluation of other organs and tissues in addition to the implantation site. Biological materials must be evaluated to ensure no transmission of AIDS, hepatitis viruses, and other diseases.

Chemical Characterization

A critical component of device safety evaluation is an analysis of the likelihood that an adverse health effect could result from exposure to materials from which the device is made. When focused on toxic effects, this analysis is known as a materials toxicity risk assessment. The purpose of toxicity studies is to identify the nature of the toxic effect produced by a chemical substance and the range of doses over which the effect is produced. A materials toxicity risk assessment can be based on an adequate chemical characterization of the device materials, characterization of the toxicity of those materials or chemicals, and information regarding exposure to the constituent materials in the course of use of the device. A chemical must reach a target tissue and be maintained at a sufficient concentration for a sufficient time in order for an adverse effect to occur. Toxicity is related to target tissue dose and, ideally, measures of such doses would be used in conducting a materials toxicity risk assessment.

The requirement for a materials toxicity risk assessment is based on the assumption that some chemicals may migrate from a device and enter surrounding tissues. The exposure dose of a specific chemical from a biomaterial depends on the physicochemical properties of the compound such as solubility, molecular weight, ionic state, and octanol-water partition coefficient (P_{ow}). Chemicals having a $P_{ow} > 4$ are less likely to migrate from a biomaterial than those that are more water-soluble. Most engineered polymers, metals, and ceramics used in medical devices are water insoluble. Thus, the chemicals subject to migration and causing cytotoxicity are the low molecular weight molecules, additives, and their reaction byproducts that have a $P_{ow} < 4$. When testing a solid sample, those chemicals on the surface of the material are the first to

Table 2.2. International standards for medical devices

Reference	Title
ISO 10993-1	Evaluation and testing
ISO 10993-2	Animal protection requirements
ISO 10993-3	Tests for genotoxicity, carcinogenicity, and reproductive toxicity
ISO 10993-4	Selection of tests for interactions with blood
ISO 10993-5	Tests for in vitro cytotoxicity
ISO 10993-6	Tests for local effects after implantation
ISO 10993-7	Ethylene oxide sterilization residuals
ISO 10993-8	Guidance on the selection and qualification of reference materials for biological tests
ISO 10993-9	Framework for the identification and quantification of potential degradation products
ISO 10993-10	Tests for irritation and delayed type hypersensitivity
ISO 10993-11	Tests for systemic toxicity
ISO 10993-12	Sample preparation and reference materials
ISO 10993-13	Identification and quantification of degradation products from polymers
ISO 10993-14	Identification and quantification of degradation products from ceramics
ISO 10993-15	Identification and quantification of degradation products from metals and alloys
ISO 10993-16	Toxicokinetic study design for degradation products and leachables from medical devices
ISO 10993-17	Methods for the establishment of allowable limits for leachable substances using health-based risk assessment
ISO 10993-18	Chemical characterization of materials
ISO 14155	Clinical investigation of medical devices

most likely partition into the environment; chemicals from the bulk phase of the material may migrate to the surface over time (Fig. 2.1). The actual bioavailability depends on both migration and partitioning between the material and the solvent (Fig. 2.2). In general, the amount of extractable chemical (extractable pool) is less than the total pool determined by complete dissolution of a material. This is because physicochemical factors as well as migration and partitioning affect the extractable pool. The kinetics or rate of extraction will vary with the temperature and solvent or environment. Once a substance enters the body, it will be distributed by normal biological processes to various body sites, dependent on its physical and chemical properties, such as solubility, polarity and molecular weight.

Guidances and standards for chemical characterization of medical devices are the direct response to these concerns. ISO addressed this issue in parts 9, 13, 14, and 15 (Table 2.2). These documents include a general technical report (part 9) and three standards on in vitro extraction studies of polymeric, metallic, and ceramic materials. The vascular graft guidance recommends extraction with solvents of varying polarities including dichloromethane and ethanol/saline solutions (FDA, 1993).

CDRH has advanced these standards by linking chemical characterization with hazard and risk assessment (Fig. 2.3). The physical/chemical characterization of the material(s) generates a list of potential leachable materials used in manufacturing and sterilization. This list

Table 2.3. Biological evaluation tests for consideration

Device Categories			Biological Effect							
Body Contact	Category Contact	Contact Duration (see footnote)	Cytotoxicity	Sensitization	Irritation or Intracutaneous Reactivity	Systemic Toxicity (Acute)	Subchronic Toxicity (Subacute Toxicity)	Genotoxicity	Implantation	Hemocompatibility
Surface Devices	Skin	A	X	X	X					
		B	X	X	X					
		C	X	X	X					
	Mucosal membranes	A	X	X	X	O				
		B	X	X	X	O	O		O	
		C	X	X	X	O	X		O	
	Breached compromised surfaces	A	X	X	X	O				
		B	X	X	X	O	O			
		C	X	X	X	O	X	X	O	
External Communicating Device	Blood path, indirect	A	X	X	X	X				X
		B	X	X		X	O			X
		C	X	X	X	X	X	X	O	X
	Tissue,[§] bone or dentin	A	X	X		O				
		B	X	X	O	O	O	X	X	
		C	X	X	O	O	O	X	X	
	Circulating blood	A	X	X	X	X		O		X
		B	X	X	X	X	O	X	O	X
		C	X	X	X	X	X	X	O	X

continued on next page

***Table 2.3. Biological evaluation tests for consideration** (continued)*

Device Categories			Biological Effect							
Body Contact	**Category Contact**	**Contact Duration (see footnote)**	**Cytotoxicity**	**Sensitization**	**Irritation or Intracutaneous Reactivity**	**Systemic Toxicity (Acute)**	**Subchronic Toxicity (Subacute Toxicity)**	**Genotoxicity**	**Implantation**	**Hemocompatibility**
Implant Devices	Tissue[§] or bone	A	X	X	X	O				
		B	X	X	O	O	O	X	X	
		C	X	X	O	O	O	X	X	
	Blood	A	X	X	X	X			X	X
		B	X	X	X	X	O	X	X	X
		C	X	X	X	X	X	X	X	X

Contact duration: A, limited (<24 hour); B, prolonged (24 hour to 30 days); C, permanent (> 30 days)
X: From ISO 10993-1: Biological evaluation of medical devicesæPart 1: Evaluation and testing.
O: Additional recommendations of the U.S. Food and Drug Administration, Bluebook Memorandum G-1, 1995.
[§] Tissue includes tissue fluids and subcutaneous spaces

Table 2.4. Supplementary evaluation tests for consideration

Device Categories			Biological Effect			
Body Contact	**Category Contact**	**Contact Duration (see footnote)**	**Chronic Toxicity**	**Carcino-genicity**	**Reproductive or Develop-mental Effects**	**Biodegra-dation**
Surface Devices	Skin	A				
		B				
		C				
	Mucosal membranes	A				
		B				
		C	O			
	Breached compromised surfaces	A				
		B				
		C	O			
External Communica-ting Device	Blood path, indirect	A				
		B				
		C	X	X		
	Tissue, bone or dentin	A				
		B				
		C		X		
	Circulating blood	A				
		B				
		C	X	X		
Implant Devices	Tissue or bone	A				
		B				
		C	X	X		
	Blood	A				
		B				
		C	X	X		

Contact duration: A, limited (< 24 hour); B, prolonged (24 hour to 30 days); C, permanent (> 30 days)
X: From ISO 10993-1: Biological evaluation of medical devices—Part 1: Evaluation and testing.
O: Additional recommendations of the U.S. Food and Drug Administration, Bluebook Memorandum G-1, 1995.
§ Tissue includes tissue fluids and subcutaneous spaces

presumes that all constituent materials of the device are bioavailable and would include the characterization of the chemicals used and products formed in the manufacturing, processing, and sterilization of the medical device; materials of synthesis; contaminants such as unreacted monomers; and additives, and their byproducts, if any. The guidance also recognizes that under conditions of use, device materials may undergo degradation, which may result in the production of additional chemical species (i.e., byproducts), the potential toxicity of which must be considered. This characterization is used to develop protocols of solubility, extraction techniques, and analyses of monomers, oligomers and copolymer composition, and other extractives. Then, the patient exposure is estimated, i.e., the extent, if any, that the chemicals and degradation products will be bioavailable. A default assumption of 100% bioavailable may be used in lieu of a scientifically based estimate or measurement. In place of assuming 100% bioavailability, the material may be extracted under conditions that maximize extraction efficiency and minimize

Table 2.5. Principles for the evaluation of medical devices*

1. The selection and evaluation of any material or device intended for use in humans requires a structured program of assessment. In the design process, an informed decision shall be made and documented that weighs the advantages/disadvantages of the various material and test procedure choices. To give assurance that the final product will perform as intended and be safe for human use, the program shall include a biological evaluation. The biological evaluation shall be planned, carried out, and documented by knowledgeable and experienced individuals capable of making informed decisions based on the advantages and disadvantages of the various materials and test procedures available.
2. In the selection of materials to be used in device manufacture, the first consideration should be fitness for purpose having regard to the characteristics and properties of the material, which include chemical, toxicological, physical, electrical, morphological and mechanical properties.
3. The following should be considered for their relevance to the overall biological evaluation of the device: a) the material(s) of manufacture; b) intended additives, process contaminants, and residues; c) leachable substances; d) degradation products; e) other components and their interactions in the final product; and f) the properties and characteristics of the final product.
4. Tests and their interpretation to be used in the biological evaluation should take into account the chemical composition of the materials including the conditions of exposure as well as the nature, degree, frequency, and duration of the device or its constituents to the body.
5. All potential biological hazards should be considered for every material and final product but this does not imply that testing for all potential hazards will be necessary or practical.
6. Any in vitro or in vivo tests shall be based on end-use applications and appropriate good laboratory practice followed by evaluation by competent informed persons. Whenever possible, in vitro screening should be carried out before in vivo tests are commenced. Test data, complete to the extent that an independent analysis could be made, shall be retained.
7. The materials or final product shall be considered for biological re-evaluation if any of the following occurs: a) any change in the source or in the specification of the materials used in the manufacture of the product; b) any change in the formulation, processing, primary packaging, or sterilization of the product; c) any change in the final product during storage; d) any change in the intended use of the product; and e) any evidence that the product may produce adverse effects when used in humans.
8. The biological evaluation performed in accordance with this part of ISO 10993 should be considered in conjunction with the nature and mobility of the ingredients in the materials used to manufacture the device and other information, other nonclinical tests, clinical studies, and post-market experiences for an overall assessment.

*From ISO 10993-1.

decomposition of extractants and artificial decomposition of the material. A counterproposal recommending analysis only of "chemicals of concern" based on physical/chemical characterization of a material is being considered. A chemical of concern is defined as any leachable chemical that may be present in significant amounts (> 0.1% in the material) or is of a class of chemicals with a potential to create potent biological hazards. After the chemical analyses, identified and quantified extractants are assessed for potential biological hazards as used in the final device at the levels determined to be present in the material, and if appropriate, at their rates of migration from the material. This information is compiled to define the exposure dose and risk of adverse effects of the extractive chemicals from the material or medical device.

Compounds that are predicted to be bioavailable in quantities greater than the proposed thresholds for systemic toxicity should be experimentally quantified using extraction conditions simulating normal use of the device. Partial identification may be sufficient only if the

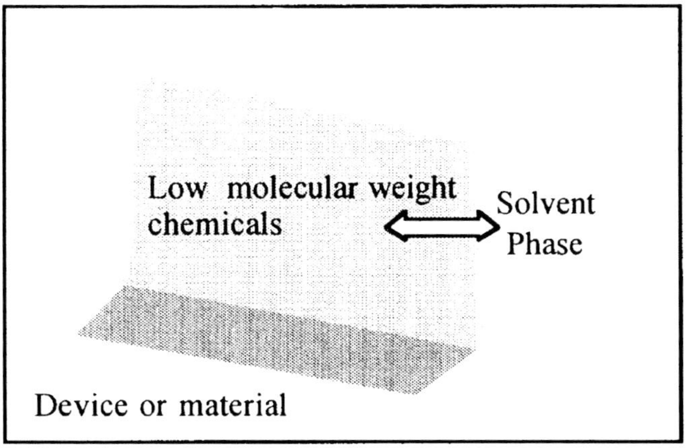

Fig. 2.1. Partitioning and migration of extractables into solvent.

constituent represents a group of compounds that are considered relatively nontoxic based on their chemical structure. For example, the total quantity of oligomers extracted from a polymeric material may substitute for identification and quantitation of each dimer, trimer, tetramer, and so forth. The U.S. Pharmacopeia monograph on container bottles made of polyethylene terephthalate is an example of use of total amount of extractable oligomers (i.e., total terephthaloyl moieties) rather than quantification of individual chemicals (U.S. Pharmacopeia, general Chapter <661> Containers). The final step is to link the dose of each leachable and degradation product with an assessment of the potential biological effects, viz., risk assessment. In the special case where the risk assessment results in a possible hazard, the assessment may be re-evaluated using the kinetic rate of release of the chemical.

Risk Assessment

There are three principal objectives for performing biocompatibility studies of products to which humans may be exposed: (1) spectrum of toxicity; (2) extrapolation, and (3) safety. The spectrum of toxicity seeks to determine the adverse effects of chemicals or articles and a description of the dose-effect relationship over a broad range of doses. The term 'dose-effect relationship' means a biological gradient of responses in relation the size of the dose. This may include variations in response, such as susceptibility based on gender or age. Extrapolation predicts the adverse effects in other species, particularly humans. Safety is the practical certainty that adverse effects or injury will not result from exposure to a material when used in the quantity and the manner proposed for its use. With our increasing knowledge of statistics, safety is more often expressed as a calculation of probability of an adverse effect, i.e., risk.

The elements of a dossier on the safety or hazard potential of a medical device and its materials of construction includes data on single dose toxicity, repeated dose toxicity, chronic toxicity, carcinogenicity, genotoxicity, reproductive toxicity, pharmacokinetics, and special toxicity, as appropriate. The latter comprises toxicity assays of specific biological endpoints, for example, immunotoxicity, local effects, blood compatibility or neurotoxicity. There are three major assumptions in this approach that can be the source of device failure. First, the identity, quantity, or biological reactivity of the individual chemicals being extracted is seldom known. Second, there is an assumption that the biological assays are sufficiently sensitive to detect any significant adverse effects. Third, there is an assumption that the extraction in vitro under static conditions simulates the physiological degradation in vivo under conditions of, for example, stress, strain, phagocytic cells, and tissue remodeling.

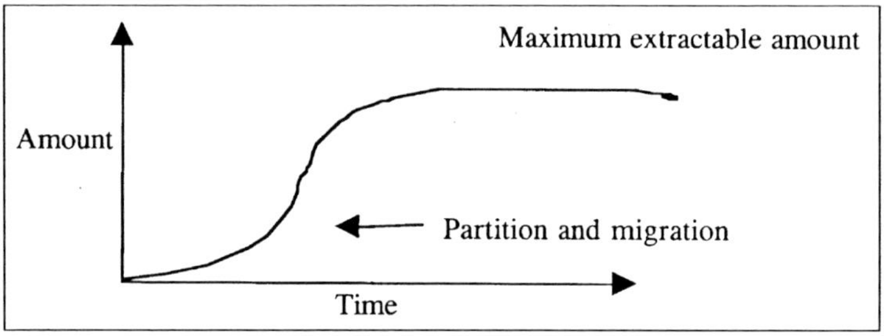

Fig. 2.2. Kinetic rate of partitioning and migration.

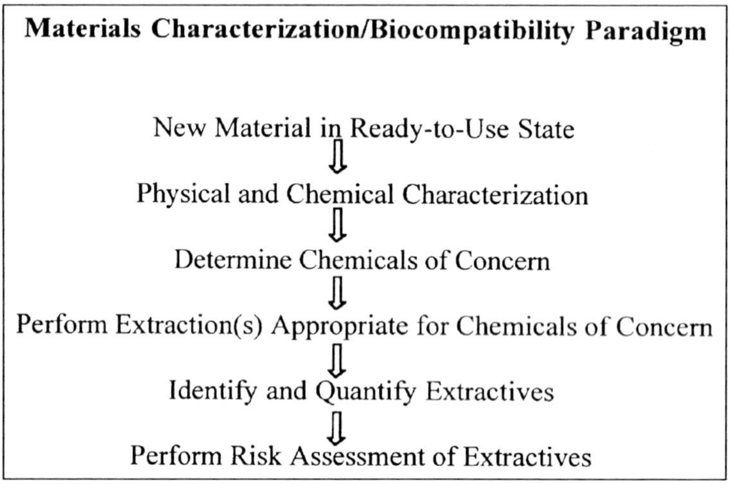

Fig. 2.3. Chemical characterization and risk assessment.

Figure 2.4 shows the elements of risk assessment that are used to assess the risk of adverse effects of the extractive chemicals and the material or medical device. Hazard identification entails identification of the specific chemicals that are suspected to pose health hazards, quantification of the concentrations present, a description of the specific forms of toxicity, and an evaluation of the conditions under which toxicity might be expressed in exposed humans. Hazard assessment equates to toxicity tests on individual chemicals, mixtures, or biocompatibility testing of the finished device or materials. Exposure assessment is the definition of route, frequency, and duration of exposure to individual leachable chemicals. Exposure assessment determines how an individual is likely to come in contact with a chemical, the amount of the chemical, and the toxic effects of the substance. This would include the route (oral, inhalation, dermal, or parenteral tissues), the rate (quantity per unit time), and the duration of exposure. Risk assessment compares the type of biological hazard with the exposure to determine the probability of an adverse effect and the likely consequences should an adverse effect occur.

In the risk characterization and assessment phase, the estimated dose of each device constituent received by the patient is compared to the respective levels of the constituents that produce various adverse biological effects or to protective health-based exposure levels derived from information on the biological effects of the chemical constituent. Biological effects include, for example, local effects, systemic toxicity, carcinogenicity, pyrogenicity, and other biological endpoints. If the dose of the constituent received by the patient is less than the dose of the compound(s) shown to produce adverse effects, then it can be predicted that adverse biological effects are unlikely to occur in patients exposed to the device. In risk assessment, apples are compared with apples. That is, acute biological effects are compared with acute exposures, chronic effects with chronic exposures. Risk assessment may result in either qualitative or quantitative outcomes depending on the nature of the input data. Most materials and finished medical devices produce no observable adverse effect when tested at the physiological or anatomical limits of the in vitro and animal models used in nonclinical evaluations. Therefore, the risk assessment from the animal bioassays is often qualitative. Quantitative risk assessments are used for specific extractable chemicals from the materials or medical device.

The current paradigm is to evaluate the medical device and/or portions thereof with a variety of biological assays designed to satisfy the eight elements of the dossier, as appropriate for that device. Additionally, leachable chemicals and degradation products from the medical device for the same eight elements is assessed, whenever possible (Table 2.6). The result is an iterative dossier describing the biological tests on the medical device followed by the biological effects of each extractable chemical or biodegradation product. Pharmacological effects are included in Table 2.6 because bioactive pharmaceutical substances are being incorporated into selected polymeric medical devices either in the bulk phase of the polymer or as a coating. It is not uncommon to have incomplete toxicology data for an extractable chemical among the eight bioassay categories. When this occurs, professional judgment determines whether additional studies are necessary or if structure-activity, computer modeling, and the weight of evidence from biocompatibility data, public literature, and prior clinical experience with the medical device will sufficiently answer concerns about the hazard potential.

In the past, in vitro and in vivo medical device testing has focused on descriptive results demonstrating lack of toxicity under the conditions of the experiment. This is essentially a demonstration of practical safety, which does not truly allow for a prediction of risk. Practical safety implies that the measurement(s) occurred at a dose below which a biological effect could be detected in the assay system when compared with a control or reference group (Fig. 2.5). Under these conditions, the data only permit a statement of no adverse effect rather than calculation of probabilities or extrapolation of risk below dose levels that result in measurable biological effects. In general, a toxicity study in which no adverse effects are produced does not provide useful information for evaluating toxicity potential or estimating risk. This observation is based on a basic principle of toxicology, which states that the proportion of a population experiencing an adverse effect decreases with decreasing dose. Thus, at some dose, an experiment of any practical size will lack the statistical power to detect a real difference between exposed and unexposed subjects. That is, the exposure dose is below the detection limit of the assay. Therefore, the probability of risk must be mathematically extrapolated because the biological response is essentially below the measurable dose range of the experiment. The two common models for extrapolation are linear, and nonlinear or threshold models (Fig. 2.5). The conservative, linear model is generally used in the absence of specific, mechanistic data to support a nonlinear or threshold model of extrapolation. The distinction between practical safety and statistical probability is most relevant in the context of irreversible, adverse, biological effects such as carcinogenicity, genotoxicity, and some immunological effects. In these examples, data from carcinogenicity and genotoxicity assays are used to extrapolate probabilities as low as less than one in a population of one million.

An ISO standard entitled, Methods for the Establishment of Allowable Limits for Leachable Substances using Health-based Rrisk Assessment, provides a broad overview of quantitative risk assessment (ISO 10993-17). The first step is to divide the biological effect dose by the exposure dose of extractable chemical. The quantity of extractable chemical may be that in the final device or the rate of migration from the device. The second step is to divide this result by

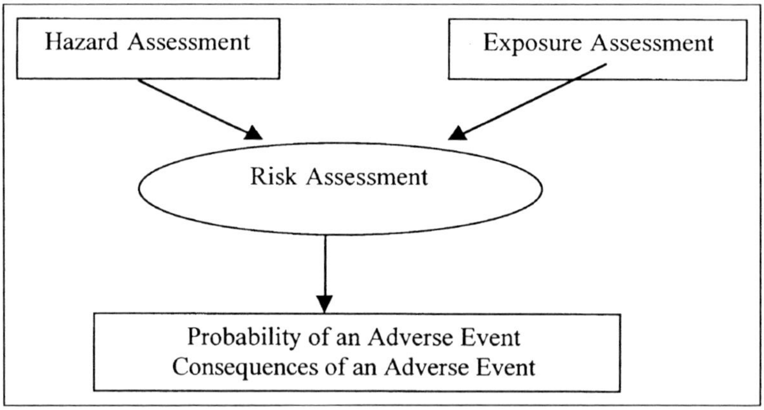

Fig. 2.4. Toxicology evaluation paradigm.

uncertainty factors for variation within species, variation across species, the quality of the data, and differences in the exposure conditions of the animal data and the predicted clinical usage. Together, these two steps are termed the safety margin approach and the result from the second division step is the 'margin of safety.' The magnitude of the uncertainty factors will depend upon the type of study being evaluated. For example, the uncertainty factor needed to calculate a margin of safety from irreversible biological effects data would be greater than the one needed from dose-dependent reversible biological effects. The general formula for calculating the margin of safety is:

$$\text{Margin of safety} = \frac{\text{Biological Effect Dose (mg/kg bw/day)}}{\text{Exposure dose (mg/kg bw/day) x uncertainty factors}}$$

Typically, high quality data from the most sensitive species are used to calculate margin of safety values. Doses causing no biological effect(s), i.e., the no-observed-effect level (NOEL) or no-observed-adverse-effect level (NOAEL), are used whenever possible. Lowest-observed-effect levels (LOELs), lowest-observed-adverse-effect levels (LOAELs), or even lowest toxic dosage (TDLo) and median lethal dosage (LD50) may be used. The exposure dose is the dividend of the amount of extractable chemical divided by the adult human bodyweight (bw) of 50-70 kg for adults, (depending on gender and ethnic group) or 10 kg for children. The selection and size of uncertainty factors used to calculate margin of safety values might be arbitrary multiples of 10 in cases where there is limited toxicological and toxicokinetic data available. That is, an uncertainty factor of 10 x 10 = 100 for variation within a species (individual variation) and between species (for example, extrapolation from rodent to humans). A third multiple of 10 may be applied to the uncertainty factor for differences in route of exposure between the device and the biological data (for example, comparison of an implanted device with oral toxicity data). This would yield a total uncertainty factor of 1,000. This default approach in the selection and size of uncertainty factors may be supplemented by more definitive data on target tissue toxicity and species differences in absorption, distribution, metabolism, and excretion of the chemical (toxicokinetics). Thus, the actual rate of exposure rather than an assumed instantaneous rate could modify the uncertainty factors. This modification is particularly appropriate for chemicals which are rapidly metabolized and excreted, and therefore, do not accumulate in the body after daily exposure. This qualitative probability is evaluated for each type of biological assay after acute, subchronic or chronic exposure. A small margin alerts the investigator to watch for adverse effects in humans such as those that were evident in the nonclinical studies. Examples of the margin of safety method are found in

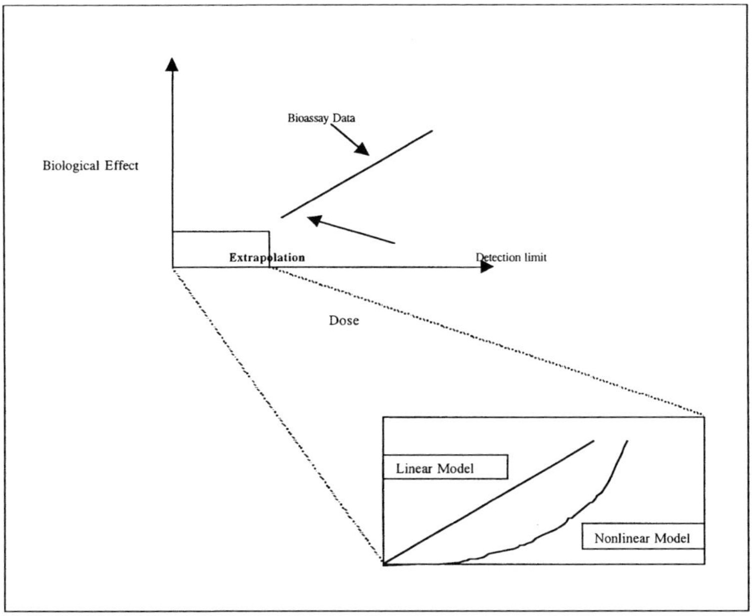

Fig. 2.5. Linear and non-linear extrapolation models.

Table 2.6. Paradigm for biological evaluation and risk assessment of medical devices

Biological Tests of Medical Device or Materials	Potential Chemical Extractives	Biological Evaluation
Cytotoxicity	Inorganic compounds	Single dose toxicity
Sensitization	Organic compounds (low molecular weight)	Repeated dose toxicity Chronic toxicity
Irritation or intracutaneous reactivity	Lubricants and processing aids	Carcinogenicity
Systemic toxicity (acute toxicity)	Antioxidants	Genotoxicity
Subchronic toxicity (subacute toxicity)	Monomers and/or oligomers	Reproductive and developmental effects
Genotoxicity	Sterilants	Pharmacokinetics
Implantation	Solvents	Special toxicity:
Hemocompatibility	Colorants	immunological effects,
Chronic toxicity	Degradation products	neurotoxicity,
Carcinogenicity	Other chemicals or byproducts	irritancy, pharmacology,
Reproductive and developmental effects		or other bioassays.
Biodegradation		

the case studies described herein and in the standard for allowable residues for ethylene oxide in medical devices (ISO 10993-7).

Case Studies of Materials Toxicity Risk Assessment

The polymer science literature identifies many low molecular weight chemicals and rearrangement products in synthetic polymers. Polymerization reactions are seldom, if ever,

100% complete. Incomplete polymerization necessitates an extraction and purification process to remove low molecular weight monomers and oligomers. The extent of this purification process and the amount of residue(s) are one of several criteria for establishing the purity grade of a polymer. Other residues may originate from additives to the polymer blend to improve the manufacturing process such as lubricants and antioxidants. The application of more extensive characterization of extractable chemicals from medical devices is visible on the horizon. Recent failures as the mammary implant, pacemaker leads, and other implantable devices have led to a FDA proposal of extractable chemicals in penile prostheses and vascular grafts. Chemical testing is also included among the criteria for establishing substantial equivalence of silicone polymers from different suppliers (Gould et al 1993). Similarly, ASTM F0748 notes, "Test selection is based upon a stable manufacturing process and for materials which have been characterized chemically...(such as gas chromatography, high performance, liquid chromatography, and atomic absorption analyses)..." The trend towards more extensive chemical characterization is not limited to implantable devices. A recent proposal appeared in Pharmacopeial Forum (Gorski, Schuette and Wallin, 1992) recommended inclusion of an isopropyl alcohol extract among the chemical assays for plastics used in pharmaceutical containers and some medical devices. This section reviews several case studies that integrate the biocompatibility, chemical characterization, and risk assessment phases of product development.

Biocompatibility

The simplest examples of the interrelationship between extractive chemicals and biological effects are those of Homsy (1970), Ikarashi, et al (1992), and Nakamura, et al (1990). Homsy prepared pseudoextracellular fluid extracts of 25 different materials, by heating at 115°C for 72 hours. The extracts were evaluated for cytotoxicity using newborn mouse heart tissue and characterized for the total amount of organic molecules. The latter were measured by infrared spectrophotometry to detect primary, secondary and tertiary carbon-hydrogen bonds and expressed as moles of n-hexanol. This analytical method was a predecessor of the current measurement of the total amount of organic carbon. The materials evaluated included nylon, polyvinyl chloride, polyurethane, polystyrene, polypropylene, and acrylobutadienestyrene. Figure 2.6 shows both low and high levels of organic carbon (expressed as n-hexanol) were associated with moderate to severe cytotoxicity ratings. The conclusion from this study is that it is the specific extractable chemical(s) rather than the total organic or inorganic chemicals that are the cause of cytotoxicity. Studies by Ikarashi, et al (1992), and Nakamura, et al (1990), illustrate directed studies to associate a toxic chemical with cytotoxicity assays. These studies tested 40 different brands of rubber gloves by in vitro cytotoxicity assays and coupled these with chemical analyses of known vulcanizing accelerators and antioxidants. The zinc dialkyldithiocarbamate chemicals were shown to be highly toxic in a colony growth assay and inhibited the growth of Chinese hamster V79 cells by 50% (50% inhibition concentration, IC50) at concentrations of 0.2-5 μg/mL. A regression equation was derived to relate the contribution of each chemical in the latex material to the cytotoxic response in vitro or in vivo using an implantation assay. The amount of chemical released under the conditions of the biological assay was not given. Thus, the relationship between the quantity of extractable dialkyldithiocarbamate and cytotoxicity rating for a given material was not clear.

Chemical Characterization

This section will illustrate the application of risk assessment to extractives from a solvent sealant and an antioxidant. The examples illustrate quantifying the amount of extractive under the predicted clinical conditions of use.

A published study on cyclohexanone in administration sets (Danielson, 1991) illustrates application of the target extractives paradigm to a solvent sealant. Cyclohexanone is the most common solvent for sealing polyvinyl chloride components of medical devices. Danielson initially tested parenteral solution administration sets for chemical leaching with methylene chloride to identify the target extractives. The capillary gas chromatograms showed two major peaks alongside minor blips (Fig. 2.7). The major peaks, which are the target extractives, were then identified. Peak A, the largest in the chromatogram, is cyclohexanone. This solvent is used as a welding agent for polyvinyl chloride and is difficult to evaporate from polyvinyl chloride because it has a high boiling point. That is, the apparent disappearance of the solvent is actually dissolution into the bulk phase of the polymer. To quantify the amount of cyclohexanone that a patient might be exposed to, filtered distilled water was drained through each administration set over 24 hours at a rate that simulated the clinical conditions of use. Danielson reported an average patient exposure of 120 micrograms of cyclohexanone from each administration set. Thus, patient exposure would be equivalent to 2 microgram/kg bw for a 60 kg patient.

The next step is to evaluate the hazard potential and patient risk to an exposure of 2 micrograms/kg bw of cyclohexanone over 24 hours. The general approach for this activity is given in the right column of Table 2.7. The main pharmacological action of cyclohexanone is central nervous system depression. The toxicological effects are highly dependent on the rate of exposure and, hence, blood concentration.

Quantitative risk assessment of selected toxicity data of cyclohexanone is shown in Table 2.7. In the example of exposure from an administration set, the gravimetric dose is compared with the toxic dose of cyclohexanone to determine the risk of adverse effects. Intravenous studies of the acute or single dose effects of cyclohexanone in the rat, dog and monkey report the lowest lethal dose is 284 mg/kg bw. This value was first divided by the exposure dose of 2 microgram/kg bw and then divided by an uncertainty factor for acute toxicity. The uncertainty factor of 100 was based on the default factors of 10 for within species and between species variability (viz., 10 x 10 = 100). This process was repeated for the 28-day intravenous toxicity study in the rat, and the 25-week and lifetime oral (drinking water) studies except that an additional uncertainty factor of 10 was applied to the oral studies. Overall, the estimated safety margin of cyclohexanone exposure from an administration set ranged between 206 and 1,420.

The estimated safety margin for cyclohexanone was refined through application of more definitive data on toxicokinetics. Studies by Koeferl et al (1981) and Martis et al (1980) showed the intravenous toxicity of cyclohexanone is dependent on the rate of intravenous exposure or blood concentration. Thus, the biological effect doses could be expressed as kinetic doses of mg/min/kg bw rather than gravimetric doses of mg/kg bw. Similarly, the human exposure dose could be averaged over 24 hours (Table 2.8). The net effect of this refinement is an increase in the safety margin or a reduction in the predicted risk. Thus, both gravimetric and kinetic dose data support a wide margin of safety for the use of cyclohexanone in solution administration sets.

Antioxidants are added to polymer formulations and function to capture free radicals. The capture of free radicals results in the transformation of the parent molecule into reaction byproducts. Figure 2.8 illustrates this reaction for Lupersol® 101 [2,5-dimethyl-di(t-butylperoxy) hexane; 1,1,4,4-tetra-methyl-tetramethylene bis(t-butyl peroxide)]. This chemical is used in food packaging and is classified as an indirect food additive in volume 21 of the U.S. Code of Federal Regulations, section 177.1520, Olefin polymers.

Lupersol 101 has been evaluated for acute toxicity in mice, rats and rabbits. It would be classified as practically nontoxic since the oral LD50 is greater than 32,000 mg/kg bw in rats. The intraperitoneal LD50 in mice is 1,700 mg/kg bw and the dermal LD50 in rabbits is 4,100 ± 1,300 mg/kg bw. Lupersol 101 has been classified as a slight skin irritant. Data gaps for assessment of hazard potential—no data on repeated dose toxicity, chronic toxicity, mutagenicity, etc.,—create concerns on the adequacy of essential information for risk assessment. Addi-

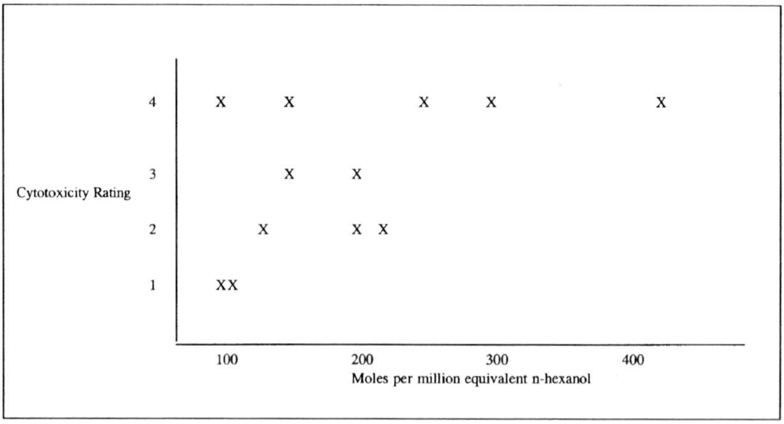

Fig. 2.6. Relationship between cytotoxicity rating and extractable organic carbon.

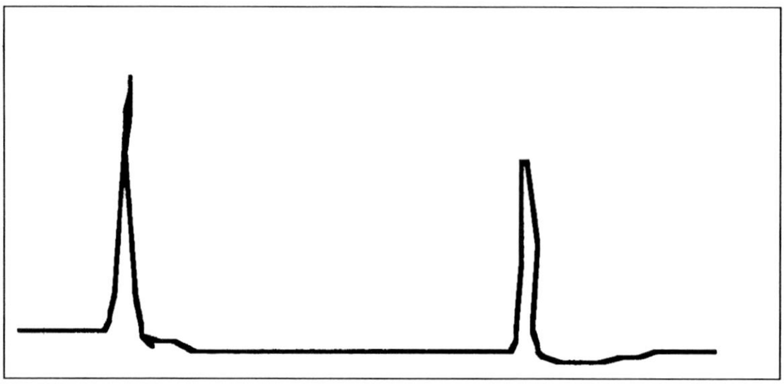

Fig. 2.7. Identification of cyclohexanone as an extractant from administration sets.

tional laboratory studies might be initiated to fill these gaps. Alternatively, toxicological data on the reaction byproducts may lessen these concerns because the ability of the body to detoxify Lupersol 101 would reduce the probability of accumulation of a toxic concentration in the target tissue(s).

Lupersol 101 is hydrolyzed at the ester bond to form t-butanol and 2,5-dimethyl-2,5-hexanediol. The rearrangement product of Lupersol 101, t-butanol, is also used as a solvent in the manufacture of antibiotics, hormones and vitamins. The limit for t-butanol in polypropylene for finished food contact articles (i.e., an indirect food additive application; 21 CFR §177.1520) is 100 mg/kg bw. t-Butanol is an indirect food additive when used in the preparation and application of coatings for paper and paperboard used as food containers (21 CFR §176.200) and in surface lubricants employed in the manufacture of metallic articles that contact food (21 CFR §178.3910). t-Butanol has anesthetic properties similar to ethanol.

The acute toxicity of t-butanol is presented in Table 2.9. Animal studies have shown t-butanol has a low potential for acute toxicity. Exposure of humans to vapors of this alcohol may induce the following symptoms: irritation of the nose, throat, and eyes, the formation of translucent vacuoles in the superficial layers of the cornea, headache, vertigo and drowsiness. Contact dermatitis, involving the fingers and hands, may occur. These effects are due to the

Table 2.7. Gravimetric safety margin for cyclohexanone exposure from a solution administration set

Toxicity Study	Biological Effect (mg/kg bw)	Biological Effect Dose Divided by the Exposure Dose	Safety Margin*
Acute toxicity, IV monkey	LDLo = 284	142,000	1,420
Repeated dose, IV rat, 28 days	NOAEL = 100	50,000	500
Repeated dose, PO rat, 25 weeks	MTD = 812	406,000	406
Chronic toxicity, PO rat and mouse	LOEL = 412	206,000	206

Abbr: IV, intravenous; PO, *per os* (oral); LDLo, Lowest lethal dose; NOAEL, no observable adverse effect level; MTD, maximum tolerated dose; LOEL, lowest observable effect level.
* Assumes an uncertainty factor of 100.

ability of t-butanol to dissolve fats and lipids from biological systems. For a safety margin of more than 100, an exposure dose of less than 0.044 mg/kg bw would be required based on the data from the LD50 in the mouse after intraperitoneal exposure, the most conservative measure of acute toxicity. Viz.,

$$\text{Exposure dose} = \frac{\text{LD50 mouse, IP}}{(\text{Safety margin})(\text{Uncertainty factors})}$$

$$\text{Exposure dose} = \frac{441}{(100)(10)(10)} = 0.044 \text{ mg/kg bw}$$

A 90-day subchronic toxicity study and 2-year carcinogenesis study of t-butanol was conducted by the US National Toxicology Program. B6C3F1 mice and Fischer 344/N rats were exposed daily to drinking water containing zero, 2.5, 5, 10, 20 and 40 mg/mL of t-butanol. The no-effect levels for direct chemical effects were 20 mg/mL in mice, 10 mg/mL in female rats and 5 mg/mL in male rats. Lethality was observed in both sexes of both species at the highest dose. Most pathological effects were secondary to starvation except for hyperplasia of the kidney transitional epithelium and inflammation of the urinary bladder in mice; and calculi, dilatation, and thickening of tissue in the kidney, ureter, and urinary bladder in rats.

In the carcinogenesis bioassay, neoplastic effects were renal tubule adenoma or carcinoma in male rats and thyroid gland follicular adenoma in female mice. Thyroid gland follicular adenoma or carcinoma occurred at a low but statistically insignificant incidence in male mice. Nonneoplastic effects were kidney hyperplasia and nephropathy in rats and follicular cell hyperplasia of the thyroid and chronic inflammation and hyperplasia of urinary bladder in mice.

The findings were interpreted as some evidence of carcinogenicity in male rats and female mice, equivocal evidence in male mice and no evidence in female rats. The biological significance of these findings is highly controversial for several reasons. There was no evidence of genotoxicity and the kidney tumors may be secondary to an accumulation of alpha-2-microglobulin and nephropathy, which is known to occur in aged male rats but not in other species. There was also a high mortality rate and t-butanol induced excretion of thyroid hormone resulted in reduced hormone half-life and thyroid hyperplasia.

The no effect level for hyperplasia in the kidneys and thyroid was used to evaluate safety margins because one of the mechanisms of nongenotoxic tumorigenesis is hyperplasia resulting in

Table 2.8. Kinetic safety margin for cyclohexanone exposure from a solution administration set

Toxicity Study	Biological Effect (mg/kg bw)	Biological Effect Dose Divided by the Exposure Dose	Safety Margin*
Acute toxicity, IV monkey	LDLo = 450	321,428,600	3×10^7
Repeated dose, IV rat, 28 days	NOAEL = 10	7,842,160	8×10^5

Abbr: IV, intravenous; LDLo, lowest lethal dose; NOAEL, no observable adverse effect level.
* Assumes an uncertainty factor of 100.

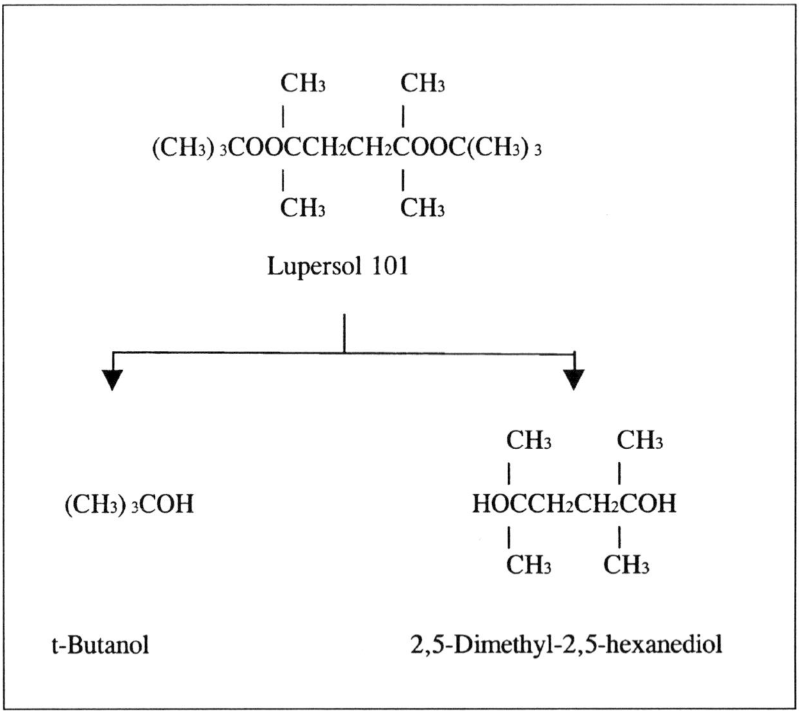

Fig. 2.8. Effect of free radicals on an antioxidant.

increased cell proliferation. The no significant effect level for kidney hyperplasia was 85 mg/kg bw in male rats. The no significant effect level for thyroid hyperplasia was 510 mg/kg bw in female mice and less than 535 mg/kg bw in male mice. Using the most conservative no significant effect level for kidney hyperplasia of 85 mg/kg bw in male rats, the exposure dose to achieve a safety margin of 200 for chronic effects is calculated to be:

$$\text{Exposure dose} = \frac{\text{(No observable adverse effect level)}}{\text{(Safety margin)(interspecies factor)(administration route factor)}}$$

$$= \frac{85 \text{ mg/kg bw (rat, PO)}}{(200)\ (10 \text{ rat to human})(10 \text{ PO to IV})} = 0.00425 \text{ mg/kg bw}$$

Table 2.9. Acute toxicity of Lupersol 101 and its re-arrangement products

Chemical	Specie	Effect (mg/kg bw)	Reference
Lupersol 101	mice, IP	LD50 = 1700	Elf Atochem
	rat, PO	LD50 > 32,000	
	rabbit, dermal	LD50 = 4100 ± 1300	
t-Butanol	mouse, IV	LD50 = 1538	Registry of Toxic Effects of Chemical Substances, Hazardous Substances Database, National Toxicology Program, and Toxline databases
	mouse, IP	LD50 = 933	
	mouse, IP	LD50 = 441	
	mouse, PO	TDLo = 103,000	
	mouse, PO	TDLo = 135,000	
	rat, PO	LD50 = 3500	
	rabbit, PO	LD50 = 3559	
	frog, parenteral	LDLo = 12,000	
2, 5-Dimethyl-2, 5-hexanediol	rat, PO	LD50 > 500	Elf Atochem
	rat, IH	LC50 > 20 mg/L	
	rabbit, dermal	LD50 > 1000	

Abbrev: IP, intraperitoneal; PO, *per os* (oral); IV intravenous; IH, inhalation; LD50, median lethal dose; TDLo, lowest toxic dose; LC50, median lethal concentration.

Oral feeding, gavage and inhalation studies showed t-butanol was toxic to maternal animals and fetotoxic, i.e., causing reductions in maternal feed intake, maternal weight gain, number of litters, litter size, and birth weights. t-Butanol was not teratogenic although delayed postnatal physiological and psychomotor performances were reported in one study.

The primary route of metabolism of t-butanol is glucuronidation and, to a lesser extent, metabolism to formaldehyde and acetone by the mixed function oxidases in liver. Induction of the mixed function oxidases (cytochrome P450) is time and dose dependent in kidney and liver. The blood half-life in rats following a single intraperitoneal dose is 9.1 hours. Repeated inhalation exposure in mice resulted in a blood half-life of less than 3 hours. t-Butanol may be excreted unchanged in the urine or following metabolism. Therefore, consideration of the biological effects of Lupersol 101 and its chemical byproducts or metabolites permit a more complete evaluation of hazard potential. This allows the user to make an informed judgment on the use of this antioxidant in a medical device application.

Biodegradation

Polymeric biodegradation products are formed primarily by chemical bond scission due to hydrolytic and/or oxidative processes in an aqueous environment. Implanted medical devices are subjected to significant degradation risk for example, from enzymes, phagocytic cells, tissue pH, and physical stresses.

During the investigations of the mammary implant failures, leachables from the devices were pinpointed as a probable cause of failure. Luu, Biles and White (1994) reported on the in vitro degradation of the polyurethane foam, Microthane® (Surgitek Corporation, Paso Robles, CA), which was used in the construction of the Meme® and Replicon® mammary prostheses. Samples of the material were extracted with phosphate buffer, pH 7.4, at 37°C with continuous, gentle stirring for 36 days. Size exclusion chromatography showed phosphate buffer extracts resulted in ten extraction and/or degradation products with molecular weights ranging from 105 to 650,000 daltons; the majority having molecular weights less than 500. The rate of leaching of 2,4- and 2,6-toluenediamine was 88 ng/g/day and 25 ng/g/day, respectively, for a total of 3 ± 0.65 mg/g and 1.13 ± 0.19 mg/g over 35 days. The design of the study, however, could not distinguish whether the extracted chemicals were residuals from the synthesis of the polymers that slowly migrated from the bulk phase of the polymer or if there indeed was hydrolysis of the polymer during the extraction period. Greater amounts of total extractable chemicals were found with more severe extraction conditions or in vivo following implantation. This study contains elements for hazard identification, for example, identification of the specific chemicals that are suspected to pose health hazards and quantitation of the concentrations present. Dose-effect assessment is obtainable from the extensive literature on 2,4- and 2,6-toluenediamine. This literature includes data on acute toxicity, repeated and chronic dose effects, mutagenicity, teratogenicity, and carcinogenicity. Exposure assessment is also available from pharmacokinetic evaluations of in vivo degradation and measurements of 2,4- and 2,6-toluenediamine in urine. With these data, it is possible to characterize the risk and determine an allowable daily exposure that would reduce the likelihood of harm in exposed people to negligible amounts. It is notable, however, that there are uncertainties and limitations of extrapolating in vitro data to in vivo conditions of biodegradation, and extrapolating animal carcinogenesis study results to humans. A subsequent clinical study of the potential for exposure to 2,4- and 2,6-toluenediamine in patients who had mammary implants confirmed that the actual release of these compounds was minimal and posed a de minimus risk (FDA, 1996).

A study by Nakamura et al (1990) is an example of a thorough analytical investigation to support clinical use of a polyetherurethane. The analyses included measurement of extractable methylene dianiline, oligomers, chemical and biological degradation studies, and biological characterization of these agents.

A third example of risk assessment is the analysis of organotin stabilizers (Mesch and Kugele, 1992). This analysis covered employee exposure during polyvinyl chloride processing, environmental effects and consumer exposure from the use or organotin-stabilized PVC in a wide variety of consumer goods from containers and blister packs for foods to pipes for transporting drinking water. Analyses of stabilizer migration were conducted in water-based, alcohol-based and fat-based food stimulants to determine the levels of migration. These levels were compared with various toxicological endpoints to quantitate the margin of safety for use of organotin stabilizers. Risk assessments are also widely used for environmental pollutants (Science and Judgment in Risk assessment).

Coating Materials

Biologically active coating materials, which are being used to improve the interface between a medical device and the biological tissues, are additional examples of the application of risk assessment. Newer generations of blood contacting medical devices are coated with ionically bonded heparin anticoagulant to reduce hemolysis. The risk assessment for these agents would evaluate the cationic surfactant and heparin separately because each component would extract at a different rate and pose different hazard potentials.

Hydrophilic coatings with antimicrobial agents such as silver chloride or organoiodines have been used on urinary catheters to reduce the incidence of infections. A risk assessment of these materials would be based on the kinetic rate of release of silver or iodine because the halide chemicals are intrinsically cytotoxic to both mammalian cells and microorganisms.

Phosphorycholine has recently been incorporated into biomaterials to enhance blood compatibility (Biocompatibles, Norfolk VA). It is a phospholipid located on the outer surface of the mammalian cell membrane and provides resistance to protein absorption. Phosphorylcholine is purported to reduce the risk of thrombotic coronary embolization by providing a hemocompatible surface for coated devices. The technology has been shown to enhance the body's acceptance of synthetic materials by effectively mimicking the biocompatibility of natural tissues. Proposed uses include guide wires, guide catheters, balloon catheters, introducer sheaths, coronary stents, vascular grafts, peripheral angioplasty products, vascular stents, heart valves, hepatic and urological stents, contact lenses, corneal implants, glucose biosensors, orthopedics, wound care devices, arterial filters, oxygenators, tubing sets and centrifugal pumps (MDDI Reports—The Gray Sheet, Jul 22, 1996, I&W4-5). The risk assessment of phosphorylcholine would focus on comparing the amount on the medical device with the endogenous concentration in human blood and tissues. Safety factors are unnecessary because the comparisons are for the same specie and tissue(s).

Pharmacologically active agents are also being added to medical devices to reduce the amount of inflammation and scar formation at the tissue interface of an implanted device. This effect is particularly beneficial for electrical stimulators such as pacemaker leads. Formation of scar tissue raises electrical impedance thereby resulting in increased current to achieve the desired electrical stimulation. Several manufacturers have marketed epicardial steroid-eluting pacing leads. The unipolar, suture-on devices contain less than 1 mg of dexamethasone sodium phosphate steroid. Steroid use reduces the acute inflammatory response typically associated with pacing leads and, thus, prevents or retards the development of higher pacing thresholds. The risk assessment of the steroid would include comparison of the rate of elution from the device and the blood levels required for pharmacological efficacy. Since the drug is only released within the first few days after implantation, the assessment would require kinetic modeling of local tissue concentrations.

Conclusion

This Chapter reviews the standards and guidelines for biocompatibility testing within the context of medical device classification and regulatory strategy. The classification of a medical device affects the nature and extent of nonclinical and clinical studies required for regulatory approval to market that medical device. This knowledge allows the manufacturer to identify an appropriate product development strategy that is consistent with the regulatory strategy. Although the guidelines for biocompatibility testing appear to be transparent, there may be additional testing requirements on the basis of historical data developed for similarly classified medical devices or individual product standards, or clinical application such as preparation of biological products, or unique drug therapy applications.

The current paradigm for biocompatibility testing includes biological assays of the medical device or materials, characterization of extractable chemicals and biodegradation products, and a materials toxicity risk assessment. The bioassays, which vary with the route and duration of exposure, include in vitro cytotoxicity, single dose and repeated dose systemic toxicity, implantation, immune sensitization, irritation, genotoxicity, and hemocompatibility. Additional bioassays of chronic toxicity, carcinogenicity, reproductive or developmental effects, and biodegradation may be required for selected medical devices.

The materials toxicity risk assessment includes a risk assessment of all constituents of the device with the assumption of 100% bioavailability. Alternatively, bioavailability may be determined by chemical analyses of the extractable substances. The chemicals are individually evaluated for toxicological effects and are then compared with the predicted exposure dose during clinical use of the medical device to derive a margin of safety for the clinical application. Case studies of a solvent, an antioxidant, and degradation products from polyetherurethane illustrated the materials characterization risk assessment process. The materials toxicity risk assessment combines identification, quantification, and risk assessment of each extractive chemical or biodegradation product.

References

1. Anon. 1992. ISO 10993-1. Biological evaluation of medical devices. Part 1. Evaluation and testing. Geneva: International Organization for Standardization.
2. Anon. 1994. Science and Judgment in Risk Assessment. Washington, DC: National Academy Press.
3. Anon. 1994. Standard F0748, Practice for selecting generic biological test methods for materials and devices. Philadelphia: American Society for Testing and Materials.
4. Anon. Guidelines for basic biological tests of medical materials and devices. Tokyo: Natl Inst Hlth Sci 1995; 191.
5. Anon. <88> Biological reactivity tests in vivo. U. S. Pharmacopeia 2000; 24:1832-1835. Rockville, MD, USA: U. S. Pharmacopeial Convention, Inc.
6. Anon. <661> Containers. U.S. Pharmacopeia 2000; 24:1930-1936. Rockville, MD, USA: U. S. Pharmacopeial Convention, Inc.
7. Danielson JW. Capillary gas chromatographic determination of cyclohexanone and 2-ethyl-1-hexanol leached from administration sets. J Assoc Off Anal Chem 1991; 74:476-478.
8. Food and Drug Administration (U.S.), Center for Devices and Radiological Health. 1986. Tripartite Biocompatibility Guidance for Medical Devices. U.S. Food and Drug Administration, Toxicology Subgroup of the Tripartite Subcommittee on Medical Devices. Rockville, MD: Food and Drug Administration, Center for Devices and Radiological Health.
9. Food and Drug Administration (U.S.), Center for Devices and Radiological Health. 1993. Guidance for the preparation of research and marketing applications for vascular graft prostheses. Rockville, MD: Food and Drug Administration, Center for Devices and Radiological Health.
10. Food and Drug Administration (U.S.), Center for Devices and Radiological Health 1994. Guidance on hemodialyzers. Rockville, MD: Food and Drug Administration, Center for Devices and Radiological Health.
11. Food and Drug Administration (U.S.), Center for Devices and Radiological Health. 1995. Required biocompatibility testing and toxicology profiles for evaluation of medical devices 5/1/95 (G95-1). Rockville, MD: Food and Drug Administration, Center for Devices and Radiological Health. [a.k.a. Blue Book Memorandum #G95-1.]
12. Freiherr, G. Advances in photodynamic therapy lure device innovators. Med Dev Diag Ind 1997; Jan:74, 76, 78-80, 82, and 84.
13. Gorski JR, Schuette MR, Wallin RF. Physicochemical Tests—Plastics: Isopropyl alcohol as an additional extractant. Pharm Forum 1992;18:4404-4407.
14. Gould JA, Liebler B, Baier R et al. Biomaterials availability: Development of a characterization strategy for interchanging silicone polymers in implantable medical devices. J Applied Biomatr 1993; 4:355-358.
15. Health Industry Manufacturers Association. Materials characterization paradigm. Correspondence of JS Benson to DB Burlington, Jul 20, 1994.
16. Homsy CA. Rapid in vitro screening of polymers for biocompatibility. J Macromol Sci-Chem 1970; A4(3):615-634.
17. Ikarashi Y, Toyoda K, Ohsawa N et al. Comparative studies by cell culture and in vivo implantation test on the toxicity of natural rubber latex materials. J Biomed Mater Res 1992; 26:339-356.
18. Koeferl MT, Miller TR, Fisher JD et al Influence of concentration and rate of intravenous administration on the toxicity of cyclohexanone in beagle dogs. Toxicol Appl Pharmacol 1981; 59:215-229.
19. Luu H-MD, Biles J, White KD. Characterization of polyester urethane degradation products. J Applied Biomaterials 1994; 5:1-7.
20. Martis LT, Tolhurst M, Koeferl T et al. Disposition kinetics of cyclohexanone in beagle dogs. Toxicol Appl Pharmacol 1980; 55:545-553.
21. Mesch KA, Kugele TG. Use of organotin stabilizers-risk assessment analysis. Ann Tech Conf Soc Plast Eng 1992; 50:1942-1945.
22. Nakamura A, Ikarashi Y, Tsuchiya T et al. Correlations among chemical constituents, cytotoxicities and tissue responses: in the case of natural rubber latex materials. Biomaterials 1990; 11:92-94.
23. Nakamura A, Kawasaki Y, Aida Y et al. Difference in tumor incidence and other tissue responses to polyetherurethanes and polydimethylsiloxane in long-term subcutaneous implantation into rats. J Biomed Mater Res 1992; 26:631-650.
24. Tang F, Huyser ES. Thermal decomposition of bifunctional peroxides. J Org Chem 1977; 42:2160-2163.

CHAPTER 3

Regulation of Medical Devices

Barry Sall

U.S. Food and Drug Administration Regulation of Medical Devices

The U.S. Food and Drug Administration (FDA) regulates all medical devices sold in the United States. As depicted in Figure 3.1, there are a variety of possible paths that a medical device manufacturer may follow in order to obtain approval or clearance to market products in the U.S. Many of the simpler, Class I, devices are excepted from the premarket review process. Most of these devices raise few, if any, biocompatability issues. The more complex Class II and Class III devices frequently include materials that closely interact with the body. In these cases, biocompatability data can make up a significant portion of the submission. Understanding FDA's concerns regarding a particular biomaterial and its application will enhance the quality of the submission, and likely accelerate the review process.

Medical Device Amendments of 1976

The 1976 Medical Device Amendments to the 1938 Food, Drug and Cosmetic Act (FDCA) gave FDA the responsibility for regulation of medical devices sold in the U.S. Not all devices are regulated in the same manner. Class I devices such as eyeglasses, tooth brushes, scalpels, prosthetic heart valve sizers and stomach pH electrodes are, for the most part, exempt from premarket review by FDA, although they can be subject to some or all quality system (QS) regulation manufacturing and development controls.

Preclinical Testing and IDEs

Preclinical testing is an integral part of the product development process. If required, much of this testing must be completed and reports available, prior to the start of human testing. 510(k) notifications for Class II devices with direct patient contact or contact with the blood supply will contain biocompatability testing data, according to ISO 10993, in order to demonstrate that the risks posed by the new device are "substantially equivalent" to the risks posed by the predicate device. Preclinical testing can also include animal and bench studies to demonstrate the effectiveness of the new device, confirm electrical safety or investigate electromagnetic interference. Although it is often prudent to discuss preclinical testing plans with FDA, no prior approvals are necessary in order to perform this testing. Both the Investigational Device Exemption (IDE)[1] and the PreMarket Approval (PMA)[2] regulations require that nonclinical laboratory studies be performed under the Good Laboratory Practices (GLP) regulations in 21CFR 58,[3] or that an explanation be provided if a study was not performed in accordance with the GLPs. Once preclinical testing has progressed to the appropriate stage, the

Biomaterials in the Design and Reliability of Medical Devices, edited by Michael N. Helmus

reports are written, overall summaries of related tests compiled and overall conclusions drawn. For relatively simple devices, conclusions of substantial equivalence may be drawn from preclinical testing alone. When complex devices are considered, preclinical testing serves as the foundation for more extensive clinical testing.

A relatively small, number of 510(k) notifications, perhaps 5%,[4] also contain human clinical data. As shown in Figure 3.1, there are two routes available in order to initiate a human clinical trial. Non Significant Risk studies involve devices that pose little risk to the study population, and can be initiated after local Institutional Review Board (IRB) review, while Significant Risk studies require submission of an IDE and IRB approval prior to study initiation. Informed Consent must be obtained from all study subjects, regardless of the risk status of the device, unless the emergency use provisions of the IDE regulations are invoked.

An IDE application contains a description of the device, theory of operation, indication for use and method of manufacture. Available preclinical data, including biocompatability information is also included in the IDE. A clinical study protocol, clinical investigator information and a clinical monitoring SOP must also be submitted. If the manufacturer plans to charge for the investigational device, this must be stated in the IDE. FDA permits recovery of research and development costs, but will not allow commercialization during the investigation. Once the IDE is received, FDA has 30 days to review the application. The FDA reviewer's main concern is to assure the level of risk incurred by the patient population is appropriate given the benefits of the investigational device. The IDE can be approved, rejected or FDA can ask for additional information before making a final determination. Typically, about 70%[5] of IDEs are approved during the first round of review. Once the IDE is approved, the manufacturer and clinical investigators must comply with a wide variety of regulations which are described in 21CFR 812. Approval of an IDE does not imply that marketing approval via the 510(k) or PMA routes is assured. It only signifies that the clinical research does not pose unreasonable risks to the study population. The manufacturer must periodically update FDA regarding the progress of the investigation.

510(k) and PMA Marketing Applications

More than 99% of all the medical devices that FDA reviews in a given year are cleared for marketing through the 510(k) PreMarket Notification process. (510(k) refers to Section 510(k) of the FDCA.) The goal of the process is to demonstrate to FDA that the new device is "substantially equivalent" to a "predicate device" which was already on the U.S. market prior to the May 28, 1976 effective date of the Medical Device Amendments. Historically, FDA has interpreted substantial equivalence in a broad sense. For an electronic device with no direct patient contact, a table containing a point-by-point comparison of key engineering features of the device is often sufficient. Class II devices such as some implants, many catheters, electrocardiograph systems and ultrasound imaging systems are all included in an intermediate risk category where 510(k) notifications and adherence to FDA Quality system regulations are required. Under the Medical Device Amendments of 1976, the submitter of a 510(k) notification could market a device 90 days after submitting the notification to FDA. As we shall see later in this chapter, the Safe Medical devices Act of 1990 made several significant changes to the 510(k) process.

Approximately 40 medical devices are approved for marketing in the U.S. through the PMA process each year. All PMA devices are Class III. The PMA process is used for devices that cannot be shown to be "substantially equivalent" to a suitable predicate device. This commonly occurs because the device utilizes a novel technology or material, or is intended for a novel indication for use. The goal of the PMA process is for the manufacturer to provide "reasonable assurance" that the new device is safe and effective. This is a higher standard than the 510(k)'s "substantial equivalence" and nearly always requires manufacturers to perform human clinical trials. Biomaterial and biocompatability concerns, as with 510(k)s, are related

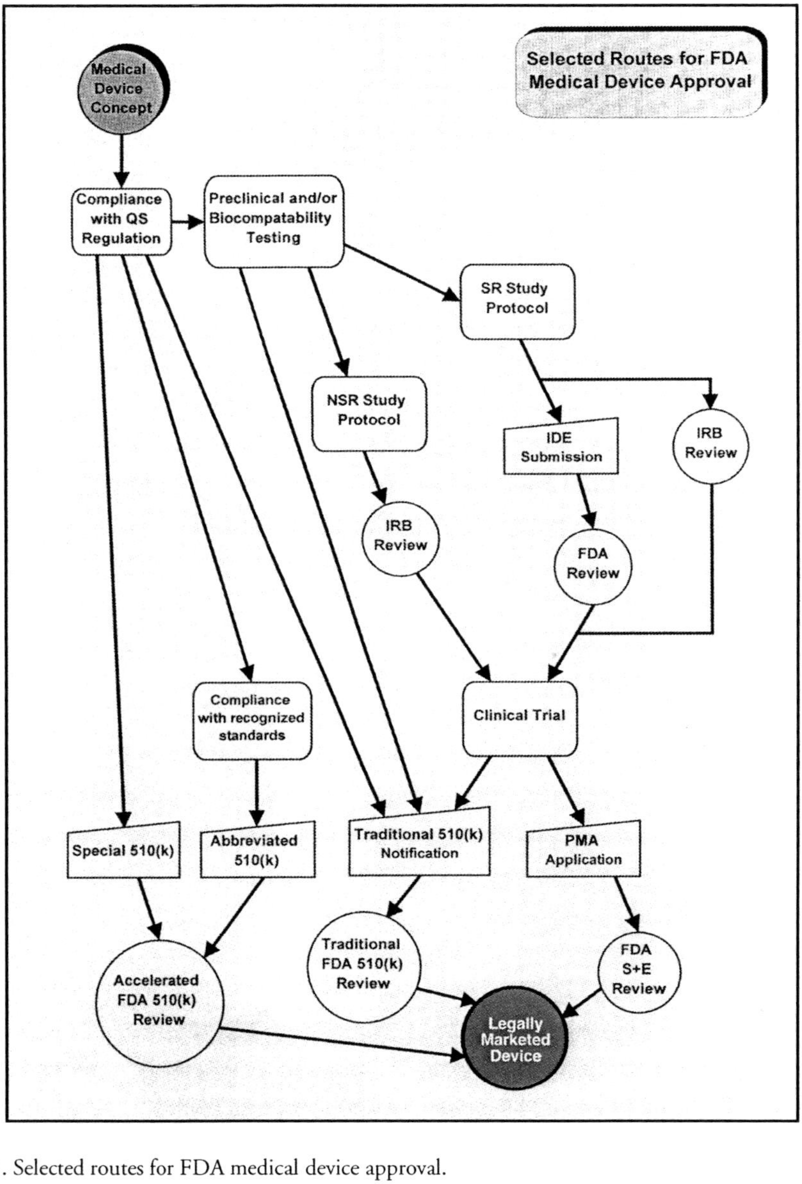

Fig. 3.1. Selected routes for FDA medical device approval.

to the type of device, materials used and the indication for use, rather than the application type. PMA review times generally extend from 9-18 months.

Quality System Regulation Requirements

The Good Manufacturing Practices regulations for medical devices becamc effective in 1978 and were the subject of a major revision, effective mid 1997. As a result of the revision, the regulation has been renamed the Quality system Regulation.[6] The purpose of this regulation is to assure that manufacturers maintain a system that can reliably design, produce, control, install and service medical devices. It is based on the international ISO 9000 standard with revisions to accommodate U.S. legal requirements. The FDA district offices, in collaboration with headquarters personnel, are responsible for enforcing these regulations by sending FDA investigators to inspect medical device manufacturers. FDA actions when noncompiling systems are identified range from documentation on the FDA form 483, warning letters and in rare instances, seizures, injunctions and civil penalties.

It is the manufacturer's responsibility to assure that the device described in the 510(k) notification or PMA is the device actually being produced. While some changes in manufacturing methodology and some substitutions of materials can be accomplished without prior FDA review,[7] the Quality system Regulation provides for controls that, among other functions, controls for changes in materials and production methods. Before any change is implemented, the manufacturer must consider if a new 510(k) notification or a PMA supplement is necessary and document that review. The Quality systems Regulations contain many other provisions, most not directly related to biomaterials. The reader is referred to the regulation and various FDA guidance documents for further information.[6,8,9]

Safe Medical Devices Act of 1990

The Safe Medical devices Act of 1990 (SMDA) [http://www.fda.gov/cdrh/ode/655.pdf] modified the 1976 Medical Device Amendments in many key areas. SMDA permits applicants to utilize any device that has been cleared through the 510(k) process as a predicate device. It is no longer necessary to select a device that was on the U.S. market prior to May 28, 1976. With regard to PMAs, SMDA makes advisory panel review optional so that the panels can focus on the most innovative technology. SMDA also contains the "four of a kind" rule which could permit submitters of the fourth PMA for a particular device to reference data submitted by the first three applicants. These data, could potentially, contain biocompatability information. As with several other provisions of this law, FDA has not drafted enabling regulations for this section and it is not currently being used. Another provision of SMDA gives FDA the ability to regulate the design process for medical devices. After considerable public comment, FDA published final regulations, which implement this provision and significantly revise all the manufacturing regulations. These changes are discussed in the following section.

Design Controls and Design History Files

The Safe Medical devices Act of 1990 (SMDA), for the first time, gave FDA the authority to regulate the design process for medical devices. Up until this time FDA investigators were limited to the examination of production and quality control records and could not review research and development documentation. The design control regulations are part of the Quality systems regulation which was fully implemented in mid 1998.

The regulation requires each manufacturer of Class II and Class III devices to implement design controls. These controls consist of a development plan applicable to the development of all new products and a Design History File (DHF) where these activities are documented. These controls are intended to regulate the design process for specific medical devices, not basic research such as the formulation and testing of novel biomaterials. A specific example may serve to clarify this distinction. If a firm is developing a polymer that may have applications for a wide variety of devices that contact the circulatory system and have other applications outside of the medical device industry, then, design controls would not apply to the development of the polymer. Once the development process for the polymer has been completed and a device manufacturer obtains supplies of this material for evaluation in a particular device, then the evaluation process is regulated under design controls. The evaluation process for biomaterials including engineering studies for functionality, durability, biocompatability and manufacturability would all be described in the DHF. Once a specific polymer has been chosen, the device manufacturer and polymer manufacturer must agree upon specifications. The regulation recommends that the device manufacturer obtain agreement from the polymer supplier that they will receive advance notification if changes are made to the polymer manufacturing process or raw materials. The polymer specification becomes part of both the Device Master Record and the Design History File. The key sections of the DHF are described below:

Design Input: Initial specifications and requirements for the device are described here. The needs of both the device user and the patient must be considered. The intended use of the device should also be included. The material that appears in the first version of this section does not have to be final and complete, but a mechanism must be in place to update the section. This section must be reviewed (signed and dated) by an appropriate individual at proper intervals.

Design Output: This section contains the results of the design effort and may include various engineering analyses as well as biocompatability data. The important feature here is that results of the design effort be quantifiable and meet or exceed previously determined specifications. It is important that all relevant design outputs be identified and included in this analysis. As with the design input section, this section must be reviewed prior to release and the reviewer's signature and date must appear on the approval page.

Design Review: A formal design review needs to occur according to a master schedule during the design process. The review team must include representatives from each functional area responsible for design activities, additional specialists, if necessary, and one individual not directly involved in the phase of the design process under review. Decisions regarding the replacement of one biomaterial with another are often made at these meetings, once the relevant data are examined. The Design history File (DHF) must document names of the participants of the design review, the version of the design reviewed, the date of the review and the results of the review.

Design Verification: This process confirms that the design output meets the specifications of the design input. The DHF must document the version of the design, verification method, date of verification and the individuals participating in the verification.

Design Validation: The device design must be validated using initial production material, not prototype units. The purpose of the validation is to ensure that the device functions according to predefined user requirements and intended uses. Devices are tested under actual or simulated use conditions. Biomaterials/biocompatability concerns, if applicable, must be addressed during this process. The entire validation process must be fully documented in the DHF.

Design Transfer: Procedures must be in place to assure that the design is correctly translated into production specifications. Raw material specifications, storage conditions and process parameters are key biomaterials issues here.

Design Changes: A change control system must be in place. This system must identify and document all changes to the device, materials and/or production methodology.

Design History File: This document must be prepared for each type of device as mentioned in the preceding paragraphs. The DHF can either be a collection of the actual documents or an index listing storage locations for those documents.

A much more detailed description of these requirements may be found in FDA guidance documents[8,9] and independently published sources.[10]

The FDA Modernization Act of 1997 (FDAMA97)

This wide-ranging law [http://www.fda.gov/cdrh/modact/modern.html] adds many features to the medical device regulatory landscape. One provision, Section 216 will permit FDA to use biocompatability data submitted in one PMA when reviewing another PMA, once the original data is at least six years old. There are also several provisions that detail various types of meetings that sponsors of IDEs or PMAs can request with FDA. This law also formalizes FDA's reliance on compliance with recognized national and international standards to expedite the 510(k) review process.

FDA Regulation of Biomaterials

The Tripartite Agreement[11]

This agreement between the U.S., Canada and the UK described a common view for the assessment of biocompatability for polymeric materials. [http://www.fda.gov/cdrh/g87-1.html] FDA officially adopted this agreement in April of 1987 and it was in effect until superseded by ISO 10993 in July of 1995. The key element to the Tripartite Agreement is a matrix that categorizes devices according to type of body contact, such as external devices on intact skin to internal devices in contact with blood; and according to the duration of contact. Duration of contact is categorized as transient (< 5 minutes), short term (5 minutes-29 days) and long term (> 29 days). Eleven tests were specified for possible inclusion in a testing program depending on the indications for use of the device. As the complexity of biomaterials technology increased and the types of biocompatability assays proliferated, FDA testing requirements strayed further from the program specified in this agreement. In addition, this agreement specifically relates to polymeric biomaterials and was never intended to address concerns for other classes of biomaterials. An April 1993 FDA guidance document provided industry with a more detailed explanation of some of the Tripartite Agreement's provisions, but made no attempt to change any of them.

ISO 10993[12]

The International Organization for Standardization's Technical Committee 194 , comprised of members from the European Committee for Standardization (CEN) and the U.S. based Association for the Advancement of Medical Instrumentation (AAMI), produced the ISO 10993 standard "Biological Evaluation of Medical devices Part 1: Evaluation and Testing" in 1994. FDA issued a memo in 1995 [http://www.fda.gov/cdrh/g951.html] that made compliance with a modified version of ISO 10993 mandatory after July 1, 1995. This document contains two tables (Refer to Figs. 3.2 and 3.3) and a flow chart (Refer to Fig. 3.4) to assist manufacturers in determining the appropriate testing plan for their device. Additional modifications to the ISO 10993 matrix which specifically relate to immunotoxicity were announced by FDA in the Immunotoxicity Testing Guidance dated May 6, 1999[http://www.fda.gov/cdrh/ost/ostggp/immunotox.pdf] The FDA modified ISO 10993 testing matrix (Refer to Fig. 3.2 and 3.3) in several specific areas.[13,14] First, for surface devices contacting mucosal membranes, acute and chronic toxicology testing along with implantation testing is expected in most cases. Second, for externally communicating devices, those that contact tissue or bone are often expected to include irritation, systemic toxicology, subchronic and chronic toxicology testing. Another important feature of the ISO 10993 standard that FDA accepted is a change in the time periods for the three exposure categories. The ISO 10993 matrix uses the contact terms "limited " (< 24 hours), "prolonged" (24 hours to 30 days) and permanent (> 30 days). The most important change here is that the limited term extends to < 24 hours, rather than the Tripartite's < 5 minutes. This permits a greater number of devices to be assessed under the simpler "limited" requirements. In documentation that accompanies the testing matrix, FDA makes the point that test selection should be based upon sound scientific reasoning. Specific biomaterials utilized for particular indications may require more or less testing than the matrix specifies. Additional, more specialized tests may also be necessary. It should be kept in mind that samples of devices used for this testing should resemble the actual marketed product as closely as possible. Devices sold as sterile should be sterilized using the method that will be used for commercial production prior to biocompatability testing. In cases where aging may affect biocompatability, devices should be aged to the end of their shelf life before testing. Organizations with internal biocompatability experts can often make these judgments independently, while other organizations frequently enlist the assistance of outside consultants and

Table 3.1. International standards for medical devices

Reference	Title
ISO 10993-1	Guidance on selection of tests
ISO 10993-2	Animal welfare requirements
ISO 10993-3	Tests for genotoxicity, carcinogenicity, and reproductive toxicity
ISO 10993-4	Selection of tests for interactions with blood
ISO 10993-5	Tests for cytotoxicity: In vitro methods
ISO 10993-6	Tests for local effects after implantation
ISO 10993-7	Ethylene oxide sterilization residuals
ISO 10993-8	Clinical investigation of medical devices
ISO 10993-9	Evaluation of biodegradation of medical devices
ISO 10993-10	Tests for irritation and sensitization
ISO 10993-11	Tests for systemic toxicity
ISO 10993-12	Sample preparation and reference materials
ISO 10993-13	Identification and quantification of degradation products from polymers
ISO 10993-14	Static test to quantify in vitro degradation of ceramics
ISO 10993-15	Identification and quantification of degradation products from metallic materials used in medical devices
ISO 10993-16	Toxicokinetic study design for degradation products and leachables
ISO 10993-17	Glutaraldehyde and formaldehyde residues in industrially sterilized medical devices
ISO 10993-18	Characterization of materials
ISO/CD 14538	Methods for the establishment of permissible limits for sterilization and process residues in medical devices using health-based risk assessment.

scientists at contract testing laboratories. Contacts with FDA prior to embarking on a time-consuming and expensive testing program are also a prudent course of action.

FDA Product Specific Guidance Documents

FDA's Center for Devices and Radiological Health (CDRH) publishes a wide variety of guidance documents to assist medical device manufacturers in determining CDRH expectations for data in marketing applications. The three best sources for obtaining any of these documents are the FDA itself. FDA maintains a World-Wide Web Site at [http://www.fda.gov] which has extensive material from CDRH. The Division of Small Manufacturer's Assistance (DSMA), at CDRH, also maintains a Facts-On-Demand service at (800) 899-0381 (in USA) or (301) 827-0100 (international). The user calls this number from a touch tone telephone and follows the automated instructions to receive a lengthy index of documents via FAX. Once the index is available, guidance documents can be ordered with a second telephone call. Finally, DSMA can be contacted directly at (800) 638-2041 (in USA) or (301) 443-6597 (international). A wide variety of private organizations provide FDA documentation for a fee. These organizations include newsletter publishers and CD-ROM publishers.

Proper Use of Guidance Documents

Guidance documents do not carry the force of law. They describe one way that industry can follow to meet FDA expectations. There may very well be many other equally acceptable paths that could be followed. When a device has one or more unique characteristics, it becomes increasingly likely that the manufacturer will need to deviate from the path described in the guidance document. These deviations should be for sound scientific reasons. In many cases,

Device Categories			Biological Effect							
Body Contact (see 4.1)		Contact duration (see 4.2) A-limited (24h) B-prolonged (24h to 30 days) C-permanent (>30days)	Cytotoxicity	Sensitization	Irritation or Intracutaneous Reactivity	System Toxicity (Acute)	Sub-chronic toxicity (sub-acute toxicity)	Genotoxicity	Implantation	Haemocompatibility
Surface devices	Skin	A	x	x	x	.	.	.	.	.
		B	x	x	x	.	.	.	.	.
		C	x	x	x	.	.	.	.	.
	Mucosal membrane	A	x	x	x	.	.	.	.	.
		B	x	x	x	o	o	.	o	.
		C	x	x	x	o	x	x	o	.
	Breached or compromised surfaces	A	x	x	x	o	.	.	.	.
		B	x	x	x	o	o	.	o	.
		C	x	x	x	o	x	x	o	.
External communicating devices	Blood path, indirect	A	x	x	x	x	.	.	.	x
		B	x	x	x	x	o	.	.	x
		C	x	x	o	x	x	x	o	x
	Tissue/bone/ dentin communicating+	A	x	x	x	o	.	.	.	.
		B	x	x	o	o	o	x	x	.
		C	x	x	o	o	o	x	x	.
	Circulating blood	A	x	x	x	x	.	o^	.	x
		B	x	x	x	x	o	x	o	x
		C	x	x	x	x	x	x	o	x
Implant devices	Tissue/ bone	A	x	x	x	o	.	.	.	.
		B	x	x	o	o	o	x	x	.
		C	x	x	o	o	o	x	x	.
	Blood	A	x	x	x	x	.	.	x	x
		B	x	x	x	x	o	x	x	x
		C	x	x	x	x	x	x	X	x

Fig. 3.2 Initial evaluation tests for consideration.
X = ISO Evaluation tests for consideration; O = Additional tests which may be applicable; Note + Tissue includes tissue fluids and subcutanous spaces; Note ^ For all devices used in extracorporial circuits; *See Figure 3.3 for Supplementary Evaluation Tests

Device Categories			Biological Effect			
Body Contact (see 4.1)		Contact duration (see 4.2) A-limited (-24h) B-prolonged (24h to 30 days) C-permanent (>30days)	Chronic Toxicity	Carcinogenicity	Reproductive/Developmental	Biodegradable
Surface devices	Skin	A	.	.	.	.
		B	.	.	.	.
		C	.	.	.	.
	Mucosal membrane	A	.	.	.	.
		B	.	.	.	.
		C	o	.	.	.
	Breached or compromised surfaces	A	.	.	.	.
		B	.	.	.	.
		C	o	.	.	.
External communicating devices	Blood path, indirect	A	.	.	.	.
		B	.	.	.	.
		C	x	x	.	.
	Tissue/bone/ dentin communicating	A	.	.	.	.
		B	.	.	.	.
		C	o	x	.	.
	Circulating blood	A	.	.	.	.
		B	.	.	.	.
		C	x	x	.	.
Implant devices	Tissue/ bone	A	.	.	.	.
		B	.	.	.	.
		C	x	x	.	.
	Blood	A	.	.	.	.
		B	.	.	.	.
		C	x	x	.	.

Fig. 3.3. Supplementary evaluation tests for consideration; X = ISO Evaluation tests for consideration; O = Additional Tests which may be applicable; *See Figure 3.2 for initial evaluation tests.

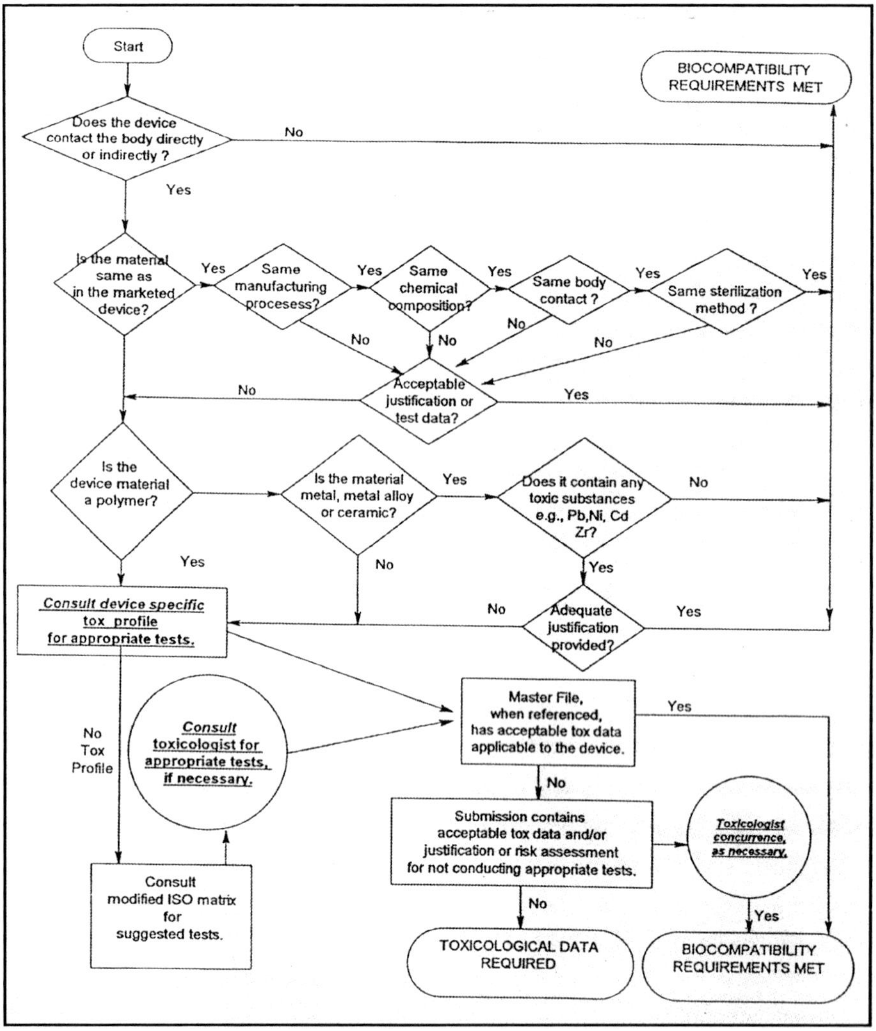

Fig. 3.4. Biocompatibility flow chart for the selection of toxicity tests for 510(k)s.

manufacturers will contact knowledgeable reviewers within the Office of Device Evaluation to obtain concurrence.

Biocompatibility Testing Program Examples

In the real world it is difficult for any guidance document or international standard to anticipate all the issues that may arise during the device development process. Device developers must utilize sound professional engineering, scientific, medical and regulatory judgement when planning a project. In some cases, going beyond the tests specified in a standard or guidance document may make both good scientific and business sense. In other cases, specific tests may be avoided if they are not scientifically justified or if the relevant data already exist. The following section contains examples of how two products that required biocompatability testing were handled. In the first case, a complicated product, used to support life was subjected to

Table 3.2. Principles for the evaluation of medical devices*

1.The selection and evaluation of any material or device intended for use in humans requires a structured program of assessment. In the design process, an informed decision shall be made and documented that weighs the advantages/disadvantages of the various material and test procedure choices. To give assurance that the final product will perform as intended and be safe for human use, the program shall include a biological evaluation. The biological evaluation shall be planned, carried out, and documented by knowledgeable and experienced individuals capable of making informed decisions based on the advantages and disadvantages of the various materials and test procedures available.

2.In the selection of materials to be used in device manufacture, the first consideration should be fitness for purpose having regard to the characteristics and properties of the material, which include chemical, toxicological, physical, electrical, morphological and mechanical properties.

3.The following should be considered for their relevance to the overall biological evaluation of the device: a) the material(s) of manufacture; b) intended additives, process contaminants, and residues; c) leachable substances; d) degradation products; e) other components and their interactions in the final product; and f) the properties and characteristics of the final product.

4.Tests and their interpretation to be used in the biological evaluation should take into account the chemical composition of the materials including the conditions of exposure as well as the nature, degree, frequency, and duration of the device or its constituents to the body.

5.All potential biological hazards should be considered for every material and final product but this does not imply that testing for all potential hazards will be necessary or practical.

6.Any in vitro or in vivo tests shall be based on end-use applications and appropriate good laboratory practice followed by evaluation by competent informed persons. Whenever possible, in vitro screening should be carried out before in vivo tests are commenced. Test data, complete to the extent that an independent analysis could be made, shall be retained.

7.The materials or final product shall be considered for biological re-evaluation if any of the following occurs: a) any change in the source or in the specification of the materials used in the manufacture of the product; b) any change in the formulation, processing, primary packaging, or sterilization of the product; c) any change in the final product during storage; d) any change in the intended use of the product; and e) any evidence that the product may produce adverse effects when used in humans.

8.The biological evaluation performed in accordance with this part of ISO 10993 should be considered in conjunction with the nature and mobility of the ingredients in the materials used to manufacture the device and other information, other non-clinical tests, clinical studies, and post-market experiences for an overall assessment.

*From ISO 10993-1.

extensive testing. The second case describes a less critical device where much of the data were obtained from previous testing programs.

Example 1: A Membrane Oxygenator

Membrane oxygenators serve as a patient's lungs when the patient is undergoing a cardiopulmonary bypass procedure. Blood flows out of the patient, into the oxygenator where carbon dioxide is removed and oxygen is added. Clearly, this device plays a critical role in

Table 3.3. Paradigm for biological evaluation and risk assessment of medical devices

Biological Tests of Medical Device or Materials	Potential Chemical Extractives	Biological Evaluation of Chemical Extractives
Cytotoxicity	Inorganic compounds	Single dose toxicity
Sensitization	Organic compounds	Repeated dose toxicity
Irritation for intracutaneous reactivity	Lubricants and processing aids	Chronic toxicity
Systemic toxicity (acute toxicity)	Antioxidants	Carcinogenicity
Subchronic toxicity (subacute toxicity)	Monomers and/or oligomers	Genotoxicity
Genotoxicity	Sterilants	Reproductive and developmental toxicity
Implantation	Solvents	Pharmacokinetics
Hemocompatibility	Colorants	Special toxicity:
Chronic toxicity	Degradation products Other chemicals or byproducts	immunological effects, neurotoxicity, irritancy, pharmacology, and other bioassays.
Carcinogenicity		
Reproductive and/or developmental effects		
Biodegradation		

keeping the patient alive. Although FDA has proposed reclassifying this device from Class III down to Class II, it currently remains a Class III 510(k) device. In January of 2000, FDA issued a revised guidance document, "Guidance for Cardiopulmonary Bypass Oxygenators 510(k) submissions" <http://www.fda.gov/cdrh/ode/1361.pdf> which provides very detailed descriptions of the biocompatability and functional testing expected for this type of device. In this particular example, the manufacturer has significantly redesigned the oxygenator, incorporating a variety of design, material and manufacturing changes.

ISO 10993 classifies this device as limited contact duration (less than 24 hours), externally communicating and circulating blood path contact. Therefore, referring to the Figure 3.2, the following tests are necessary:

Cytotoxicity, Sensitization, Irritation, Acute Systemic Toxicity, Genotoxicity and Hemocompatibility

The guidance document adds that the devices that are tested must be representative of actual production lots, utilizing the same design, materials, assembly and packaging procedures. FDA also states that the devices should be subjected to shipping tests and aged under real time or accelerated conditions to simulate the full shelf life prior to beginning testing. The manufacturer must also demonstrate that oxygenator materials are compatible with anesthetic agents and medications commonly added to the blood of bypass patients. These expectations are part of the ISO 10993 standard. This is an example of a case where it is important to refer to current guidance documents and/or contact a knowledgeable FDA reviewer in order to confirm that biocompatability testing plans are appropriate. This is especially true if the oxygenator contains any materials that are new to FDA or have not previously been used in this type of device.

Example 2: A skin electrode for monitoring cutaneous electrical activity:

This electrode is used to acquire an electrical signal that is further processed to generate diagnostic information. A 510(k) for this Class II device had previously been cleared, but included electrodes that could only be used for a few hours. The manufacturer resourced the electrode from another supplier. The new electrode could be used for not more than 24 hours. In this case, the new electrode had already been cleared for use with a therapeutic medical device, so FDA was already familiar with product, although not with its application to this particular indication. This is an especially important point. Whenever one makes regulatory judgements on a medical device, the indication for use must be clearly stated and carefully considered. A relatively small biocompatability testing program may be entirely appropriate for a device used for one indication for use, but completely inadequate for the same device or material if it is used for another, more critical indication. In this case, both indications involved placing the electrode over intact skin, so, much of the data previously gathered for the original indication of the new electrode remained applicable for its new indication. Understanding this permitted the diagnostic device manufacturer to save time and money by requesting that the electrode manufacturer provide copies of these reports so that the diagnostic device manufacturer could include them in the 510(k) Notification. Alternately, the electrode manufacturer could include these reports in a Device Master File (MAF) that is filed with FDA. The electrode manufacturer then provides its customers with letters authorizing them to reference the data in the MAF. The customers do not have access to these reports, so confidentiality is preserved. The tests included in the 510(k) were Cytotoxicity, Sensitization, Irritation and Acute Systemic Toxicity.

Even though no new biocompatability testing was required in this case, other preclinical testing was necessary. As part of the Design Control process, the diagnostic device manufacturer needed to assure that the electrical characteristics of the system were within limits during the entire recommended use period. Shelf life was another issue that required testing. The therapeutic indication utilized quite different electrical characteristics than the diagnostic indication, so the testing conducted for the original shelf life contained quite different test methods and specifications. Because of this, even though the packaging remained the same, the shelf life study was repeated using entirely different test methodology and specifications.

FDA Regulation of the Biomaterials Testing Process

In the previous sections FDA data requirements have been discussed. We have answered the question, "What tests do we need to conduct?" In this section, we address the question, "How is the recommended testing conducted?"

Description of GLP Regulations

Safety testing data such as biocompatability data are vital components to the marketing application. In order to assure that these data actually represent the true experimental results, FDA regulates safety testing with the Good Laboratory Practices (GLP) regulations (21CFR 58).[3] The regulation requires documented controls for the regulation of organization and personnel, facilities, equipment, testing facilities operation, test and control articles and study protocols.

One key provision of the regulation is the establishment of a Quality Control Unit (QAU) which periodically and independently monitors GLP-regulated studies. Just as FDA investigators can inspect manufacturer's facilities, GLP laboratory facilities are also subject to on-site inspections by FDA. When choosing a contract testing laboratory it is important to select one with a good compliance history. In extreme cases, FDA has refused to review data from a particular laboratory because of a high level of noncompliance with the GLP regulations. Careful selection of contract testing laboratories, periodic auditing and maintenance of open communication channels will reduce the likelihood of compliance issues.

Examples of GLP Noncompliance Taken From FDA Warning Letters

From time to time, inspections of GLP regulated testing laboratories result in the issuance of a warning letter to laboratory management detailing apparently serious violations of regulations. These publicly available documents list the major violations found and may include sanctions against the laboratory including disallowal of study data. One must always bear in mind that warning letters are written to prove a point and additional data may change initial FDA conclusions. The following excerpts from FDA warning letters, for medical device studies, serve to illustrate the GLP compliance areas that FDA considers important.

The Quality Assurance Unit:

"Failure to establish a Quality Assurance Unit to monitor each nonclinical study and to assure that the facilities, equipment, personnel, methods, practices, records, and controls are in conformance with applicable regulations as required in 21 CFR 58.29(b), 58.31, and 58.35. The testing facility management failed to assure that:

- the facility has an impartial and independent Quality Assurance Unit (QAU);
- test articles, study documents, raw data, and specimens are maintained in accordance with 21 CFR 58.190;
- all study personnel are knowledgeable of their responsibilities;
- deviations from these regulations were corrected and documentation of the corrections was maintained...

The Quality Assurance Unit failed to have a master schedule sheet in accordance with 21 CFR 58.35(b)(1)."

Training for Study Personnel

"Failure to have documentation to show that each individual participating or auditing this study had received any training in GLP's or that this facility provided GLP training as required by 21 CFR 58.29(a)(b).

The testing facility management failed to assure that the personnel followed the current written standard operating procedures entitled, "[purged text] Biomedical Research Standard Operating Procedures," dated September 30, 1997. For example, in Study [purged word] the testing facility failed to have current training summaries for each person involved in the study and documentation defining the critical phases and associated QAU audit schedule."

SOPs for Study Activities

"Failure to have written standard operating procedures established, during the period of this study, e.g., animal room preparation, test systems observations, data handling, storage and retrieval, laboratory test and the housing, feeding, handling and care of the animals as required by 21 CFR 58.81(b)(1-12).

There were no written procedures available for the receipt, security, storage, maintenance, disposition, or inventory control of test articles; for laboratory tests, such as blood chemistry, urinalysis, and histological analysis; for specimen collection and labeling requirements; for histopathology; and for specimen archiving."

Study Protocol

"Protocol was inadequate in that it did not clearly indicate all methods for conduct of the study as follows: (a) the model number of the control leads was not stated; the source of the dogs was not identified; the description of the diet was not included and did not address interfering contaminants; study methods to be used were not described, 21 CFR 58.120.

You failed to include in the final report the statistical methods for analyzing the data; the source of the dogs and the location of where the calibration and maintenance records for the test equipment are to be stored as required by 21 CFR 58.185.

Failure to have written documentation as required by 21 CFR 58.90(c) to show that using dog No. 714, on a previous study using a J lead and a ventricular lead, would not interfere with the dog's heart accepting the control lead.

Failure to maintain records as required by 21 CFR 58.130(e). For example: records not dated or initialed; raw data not recorded; changes not properly documented; records not recorded in ink; and records do not explain why some dogs had two sets of data or partial data collected on the same day, dog Nos. 714, 792, 745.

Specimens were not identified in a manner to preclude error in the recording of data. For example, specimens from Study [purged word] were labeled [purged text] with no other information to correlate specimens to test systems.

All data generated during the conduct of these nonclinical laboratory studies were not prepared and documented as required by this regulation. In Study [purged word] inappropriate changes were noted in data entries, such as obscuring entries in animal care charts and other records. The reasons for these changes were not documented. Also, some records associated with the study were not dated and signed by the person responsible for direct data input."

Key GLP Compliance Points to Consider When Reviewing GLP Studies

As the points included above illustrate, documentation is a key component of all GLP systems. All tasks required by regulations must be documented or FDA will assume that they were not performed.

The Quality Assurance Unit (QAU) receives a great deal of attention during an FDA inspection as the first few items in this list indicate. QAU personnel must be trained, have adequate time and be knowledgeable enough to perform their review functions assuring that study protocols and laboratory SOPs are followed. There must be enough people in the QAU so that each study can be controlled in an adequate manner. The Standard Operating Procedures (SOPs) for the QAU must describe an appropriate QA system in a sufficient level of detail. Audit reports and logs must also be carefully maintained. When testing follows internationally recognized standards, the laboratory must have current copies of those standards and their procedures must accurately reflect requirements in the standards.

Study protocols must be carefully drafted to fully describe the research effort, all test article used, number and types of animals used and their diet and all other related study procedures. It is especially important in surgical implant studies to carefully describe the location and method for placing the device into position.

Data processing and data management usually occur during or at the end of most studies and can sometimes be given less attention than the portions of the study protocol that directly relate to handling or observation of the device. No matter how well these earlier parts of the study are executed, the raw data only gain full credibility after the analysis phase of the study. These concerns begin when raw data are initially entered into study notebooks or electronic files and continue when data are placed into databases for statistical analysis.

General laboratory systems are also regulated. In order to generate credible data, laboratory equipment from electronic balances to spectrophotometers must be properly maintained and regularly calibrated. Of course, all these activities must be documented.

Validation of laboratory methods and equipment can often become an issue with GLP studies. Assays performed exactly as they are specified in the USP or standard AOAC methods do not need to be validated. If, on the other hand, an assay from the research literature is utilized, or a special purpose assay is developed, then validation becomes necessary. The validation process provides assurance that the assay accurately and reproducibly measures the parameter of interest under all expected conditions and using defined test equipment.[15-17] Of course, there must also be assurance that the parameter measured does indeed reflect the condition monitored. If the analysis method should change, revalidation may be necessary. Calibration, as mentioned above, is an important part of laboratory operations, but it is not a substitute for validation. A properly calibrated instrument can generate highly accurate, but irrelevant, data if the overall assay method is flawed.

Electronic data capture, analysis and storage is becoming widespread in all areas of biomaterials testing. These types of software offer analytical capabilities that were previously unavailable and save considerable quantities of time. As with assay methodology, software that manipulates data must be validated. Often, vendors of software specifically designed for the GLP environment will perform validations and have a mechanism in place to make the results available to regulatory authorities, if requested. Software which is well known to the regulators such as Lotus 1-2-3 or Excel do not, in general, need to be validated. However, if a researcher writes a macro using a spreadsheet, the user-defined macro must be validated to assure that it processed data in the expected manner.

The Federal Register Notices can be found on [http://www.access.gpo.gov/su_docs/aces/aces140.html]

Electronic data storage presents other challenges. Well run paper based systems provide for audit trails when data must be corrected. These notations enable a reviewer to immediately learn who made the change, when it was made and what the previous value was. This audit trail capability must be present in electronic systems. The system must be validated to assure that data cannot be changed with an audit trail being created and that all other data remains undisturbed. System security issues such as assuring that only authorized personnel have data modification privileges must also be validated. The FDA Electronic Signature Regulation (21CFR 11) contains the regulatory requirements for these systems. Electronic data management systems can save enormous quantities of time in the testing lab, however, measures must be take to assure that they perform only as intended.

Conclusion

Biomaterials involve a wide variety of regulatory issues throughout the product life cycle. Recent changes in regulations have focused an increased level of attention on the design phase of the device development process. This attention originates both from the U.S. FDA, in the form of the Quality system Regulations, and internationally from the ISO 10993 standards. Awareness of regulatory requirements and informal expectations early in the planning process can speed the entire development process, allowing the general population rapid access to innovative technology.

Acknowledgment

The author wishes to thank Ms. Angela Rogers, Regulatory Associate II, PAREXEL International Corp., San Diego, CA for her kind assistance with this manuscript.

References

1. Food and Drug Administration, Investigational Device Exemption Regulation, 21CFR 812, April 1, 2001.
2. Food and Drug Administration, PreMarket Approval Regulation, 21CFR 814, April 1, 2001.
3. Food and Drug Administration, Good Laboratory Practices Regulation, 21CFR 58, April 1, 2001.
4. Food and Drug Administration, Financial Disclosure by Clinical Investigators, Federal Register. February 2, 1998; 63:(251):72171-72181.*
5. Food and Drug Administration, Center for Devices and Radiologic Health, Office of Device Evaluation, Fiscal Year 1998 Annual Report, 1999. [http://www.fda.gov/cdrh/ode/annrp298.pdf]
6. Food and Drug Administration, Quality System Regulation, 21CFR April 1999; 820.
7. Food and Drug Administration, Center for Devices and Radiologic Health, Office of Device Evaluation, Deciding When to Submit a 510(k) for a Change to an Existing Device, January 10, 1997. [http://www.fda.gov/cdrh/ode/510kmod.pdf]
8. Food and Drug Administration, Design Control Guidance for Medical Device Manufacturers, Federal Register. March 1996; 61(58):12075-12076.*
9. Food and Drug Administration Do It By Design; an Introduction to Human Factors in Medical devices, Federal Register March 1996; 61(58):12075-12076.*
10. Vercimak Sutton, C and C. DeSain, Meeting GMP and ISO 9001 Expectations for Product Development, PAREXEL International Corp., 1996. [http://38.15.21.244/products/books/meeting.html]
11. Food and Drug Administration, General Program Memorandum #87-1, Tripartite Biocompatability Guidance, April 24, 1987.
12. International Organization for Standardization, Biological Safety Testing for Medical Devices, DIS 10993, 1993.
13. Food and Drug Administration, General Program Memorandum #G95-1, Use of International Standard ISO-10993, "Biological Evaluation of Medical Devices Part 1: Evaluation and Testing, May 1, 1995. http://www.fda.gov/cdrh/g951.html
14. Food and Drug Administration, Draft Immunotoxicity Testing Framework, October 21, 1996.
15. Food and Drug Administration, Federal Register, International Conference on Harmonisation; Guideline on Validation of Analytical Procedures: Definitions and Terminology; Availability, March 1, 1995; 60(40):11259-11262. The Federal Register Notices can be found on [http://www.access.gpo.gov/su_docs/aces/aces140.html]
16. Food and Drug Administration, Federal Register, International Conference on Harmonisation; Draft Guideline on the Validation of Analytical Procedures: Methodology; Availability, March 7, 1996; 61(46):9315-9319. The Federal Register Notices can be found on [http://www.access.gpo.gov/su_docs/aces/aces140.html]
17. Food and Drug Administration, Center for Drugs and Biologics and Center for Devices and Radiologic Health, Guideline on General Principles of Process Validation, May 1987.

Chapter 4

Nonclinical Medical Device Testing

Sharon J. Northup

The goal of nonclinical evaluation is to obtain data from in vitro or in vivo studies that will support the safety and efficacy of a medical device. Medical devices are defined as "...any instrument, apparatus, appliance material or other article intended by the manufacturer to be used for human beings solely or principally for the purpose of: diagnosis, prevention, monitoring, treatment or alleviation of disease, injury, or handicap; investigation, replacement or modification of the anatomy or of a physiological process; or control of conception..." (ISO 10993-1, 1997). Additionally, the definition provides that a medical device does not achieve its principal intended action in or on the human body by pharmacological, immunological or metabolic means. Efficacy is embodied in the purpose of diagnosis, prevention, monitoring, treatment or alleviation of disease, injury or handicap. Safety essentially implies that medical devices will not have an adverse effect on humans when used as intended by the manufacturer. This chapter will provide a review of the biological assays that are commonly used to evaluate the efficacy and safety of medical devices and integrate the information derived from these assays with contemporary recommendations for assessing the potential hazards and health risks for the patient from exposure to medical devices. This chapter contains a general overview of the requirements for safety evaluation and a detailed discussion of laboratory methodologies. Efficacy is reviewed from the dual perspectives of product design and the functional aspects of the medical device.

Overview of Biocompatibility Procedures

Nonclinical testing encompasses all of the evaluations performed before human exposure to the medical device in a clinical setting. The term is most frequently used to denote in vitro and in vivo evaluation in biological systems but may also include the mechanical and physical evaluation embodied in design control. Biocompatibility evaluation of medical products intended for use by humans consists of eight broad categories of tests, viz., single dose toxicity, repeated dose toxicity, chronic toxicity, carcinogenicity, genotoxicity, reproductive toxicity, pharmacokinetics, and special toxicity. These areas are incorporated into the International Organization for Standardization (ISO) document 10993-1 Biological Evaluation of Medical devices—Part 1: Evaluation and Testing. This ISO guideline describes a series of biological assays to be performed by the manufacturer to demonstrate a particular device is safe for its intended use (see Chapter 2, Table 2.2). The biological assays for medical devices that correspond to each element are shown in Table 4.1. The actual testing recommended or required will vary with the route of exposure in humans and the duration of use. The more invasive the route of exposure or the more extensive the duration of use, the greater the number of biological tests and the longer their duration. Biocompatibility standards serve a valuable function in identifying the essential variables of a biological assay. These variables determine the scope and quality of the bioassay.

Biomaterials in the Design and Reliability of Medical Devices, edited by Michael N. Helmus

Table 4.1. Standardized methods of nonclinical biocompatibility tests

Class	ISO 10993	Other Standards Reference
Single Dose	Part 5	USP <87> Biological reactivity, in vitro (cytotoxicity).
	Part 11	USP <88> Biological reactivity, in vivo (systemic injection assay).
Repeated Dose	Part 6	USP <88> Biological reactivity, in vivo (implantation assay).
Chronic Toxicity	Part 11	OECD guideline 453.
Carcinogenicity	Part 3	OECD guideline 451 and 453.
Genotoxicity	Part 3	See Table 4.5.
Reproductive toxicity	Part 3	International Conference on Harmonization: Guideline on detection of toxicity to reproduction for medicinal products. (US) Fed. Register 1994; 59: 48746-48752.
Toxicokinetics	Part 16	International Conference on Harmonization: Guideline on repeated dose tissue distribution studies. (US) Fed. Register 1995; 60: 11274-11275.
Special Toxicity:		
Delayed Hypersensitivity	Part 10	None
Irritation	Part 10	USP <88> Biological reactivity, in vivo (irritation assay).
Hemocompatibility	Part 4	ASTM F756 Standard practice for the assessment of hemolytic properties of materials.
Pyrogenicity	Part 11	USP <151> Rabbit pyrogen assay. USP <85> *Limulus* amoebocyte lysate assay.

The scope of a bioassay may be narrowly targeted as, for example, the rabbit pyrogenicity assay measures the change in body temperature over a specific time interval. Alternatively a broad scope would evaluate many different endpoints to identify change(s) from the control groups. Important quality variables of an in vivo study include the species and strain of animals; the age, number and gender of animals; preparation of the control, test and reference articles; treatment regimen for test, control and reference groups; in-life observations; gravimetric measures as body weight, food consumption, and organ weight; frequency and type of hematology measurements; frequency and type of clinical biochemistry measurements; macroscopic and microscopic tissue evaluations; ophthalmoscopy; analyses of excreta; types of statistical analyses; and other endpoints.

The nomenclature of biological assays is derived from the frequency of exposure, duration of exposure, duration of observations for biological effects, and assumptions regarding absorption and distribution. Single dose studies are those in which the test article or an extract thereof is administered to the test system within a 24-hour period. The test system may be an intact organism or isolated cells. Thus, in vitro cytotoxicity tests and acute in vivo systemic toxicity tests are grouped as single dose toxicity studies. In both assays, the test system may potentially be exposed to the chemicals derived from either the extraction of the medical device or by assuming extraction occurs from direct exposure to the materials or device. This text classifies implantation assays as repeated dose toxicity studies because the test samples remain in contact with the tissues for days to months throughout which there could be extended release (viz., controlled delivery) of extractable chemicals or biodegradation products.

Repeated dose toxicity study is the preferred, unambiguous term used for multiple days of dosing. Often the duration of exposure is included in the title as, for example, 7-day repeated dose toxicity study. If the duration of the test is less than 90 days (3 months), then it has historically been known as a subacute or subchronic assay. The latter terms have fallen into disuse because of their ambiguity. Exposures extending beyond 10% of the lifespan of the test animal are described as chronic assays. In the case of the rodent, a bioassay lasting longer than 90 days is a chronic assay because this duration would exceed 10% of this species lifetime. Carcinogenicity bioassays are expected to last for the lifetime of the test species which would be two years in rodents but longer in dogs or primates. Application of a chemical to the skin of an animal may be described as either a single dose study or a special toxicity study for local irritation depending on whether there is an assumption of systemic absorption.

Genotoxicity tests are assays to determine effects on the nucleic acids of the genes (i.e., mutagenicity) or the chromosome (i.e., clastogenicity). Reproductive toxicity studies focus on the anatomy and function of the reproductive tissues, the reproductive cycle, mating, fecundity (number of pregnancies per number of matings), fertility (number of females conceiving per number of females exposed to fertile males), litter size and health, and the nurturing of the offspring. Teratology studies are limited to observing effects on the fetus when exposure occurs during the critical period of fetal development. Toxicokinetic studies determine the absorption, distribution, metabolism, and elimination of foreign chemicals such as chemicals identified in extraction and biodegradation studies.

Special toxicity studies commonly applied to medical devices include irritation, immunotoxicity, and hemocompatibility. The anatomic site of application such as dermal, intradermal, ocular or mucosa and the specific mucosal site (oral cavity, vagina, penis, rectum, etc.) further subclassify irritation studies. Irritation tests may be single or repeated dose exposure protocols depending on the predicted duration of exposure in humans. Immunotoxicity studies of medical devices have traditionally focused on assessing delayed contact hypersensitivity (viz., cellular immunity) by the maximization or closed patch methods. In recognition of the limitations of the hypersensitivity assay in identifying all potential effects on the immune system, the U.S. Food and Drug Administration has recently recommended additional immunoassays (Langone, 1996).

Biocompatibility assays are generally performed at the biological limits of the test system. For an in vitro assay, the biological limit is defined as the maximum dilution of the culture media components that is compatible with normal cell viability and reproduction or approximately 10% of the projected surface area of an adherent cell culture in the direct and indirect contact assays. For an in vivo biological assay, the biological limit is the volume of extract nearly equivalent to the blood volume in a systemic injection assay or the limit of a local tissue exposure site such as the size of a muscle or bone. As discussed in Chapter 2, the lack of adverse effects in biological limit assays allows an interpretation of practical safety but does not identify the hazard potential or the risk.

Sample Preparation

Sample preparation is a critical variable in the conduct of the biocompatibility assays. The preferred test sample is the intact medical device that has been processed and sterilized in the same manner as the medical device that will be used in humans. It is, however, not always practical to use the intact medical device because of the design constraints inherent in the biological test. Therefore, representative materials used in the medical device or extracts of the device or its materials of construction may be substituted. The development of standardized methods of extracting the inert, solid materials used in medical devices to meet the requirements of the bioassays permits comparison of the biocompatibility of materials being considered for use in the design of a medical device.

Sample preparation has occasionally been associated with adverse outcomes in the assessment of safety and efficacy (Stark 1996). There may be errors in sample identification, formulation errors, incorrect manufacturing processes, incomplete curing of an epoxy resin, excessive solvent residues, surface contaminants from improper handling, or improper storage conditions. These types of errors are more likely to occur in the early stages of product development programs when several similar materials are being screened or formulated and when manufacturing processes have not yet been validated. Testing two or more samples from different lots, separate manufacturing shifts, or production days may assist in confirming whether the results are associated with the sampling errors and if they are reproducible. After the reproducibility of the adverse biological effects is confirmed, further investigations of the causative agent can be initiated, if appropriate.

Extraction conditions are usually static at temperatures of 37, 50, 70, or 121°C for periods of 1 to 72 hours. Temperatures greater than body temperature were based on the heat history established by microbiologists to reduce the bioburden of laboratory equipment along with extraction studies of polymeric food containers. That is, from the historical perspective of microbiology, the conditions of extracting at 50°C for 72 hours, 70°C for 24 hours or 121°C for 1 hour were equivalent in sterilizing equipment. When these time and temperature conditions were adopted for extraction of medical devices and materials, the rationale was modified as either simulating or exaggerating the conditions of use of the product. For example, a 37°C extract of a material might simulate a product that is used at core body temperature and is never exposed to higher temperatures. Likewise, an extraction at 121°C for 1 hour might simulate a product that is subjected to autoclave sterilization.

The key assumption about extract preparation is that the wide variety of polar and nonpolar solvents and conditions will mimic the degradation and extraction that occurs in product manufacture or use. Common extractants are 0.9% saline, 5% ethanol in saline and vegetable oils. Alternatively, cell culture media and dimethyl sulfoxide may be used in the cytotoxicity and genotoxicity assays, respectively. Specific extractants may be preferred for certain types of products. Drug-delivery devices may be extracted with drug product vehicles; dental devices with artificial saliva; electrode gels with artificial perspiration; and wound dressings with pseudo-extracellular fluid or mammalian cell culture medium containing serum.

The composition of the mixture of chemicals in an extract of a medical device or material will generally follow the basic laws of chemical solubility. An aqueous solvent may contain simple acids, bases, inorganic ions, alcohols, metal catalysts, or other water soluble, mobile constituents. A nonpolar solvent may contain water insoluble compounds such as complex phenols and organic compounds that are reaction products from an antioxidant. Extracts prepared from culture media that contain serum or other proteins may permit extraction of some water insoluble, mobile constituents through the action of protein binding as well as extracting water-soluble constituents of the device.

These standardized methods for preparing extracts for bioassays should not be confused with physicochemical characterization of the materials used in a medical device. Characterization specifically denotes the identification of individual chemicals that may be extracted from a medical device rather than the mixture that is extracted with a biocompatible solvent for the standardized biocompatibility assays. FDA's guidance on vascular grafts, for example, requires materials characterization whereby solvents should be chosen that are expected to solubilize the low molecular weight migrants thus facilitating exhaustive extraction of the chemicals. Inasmuch as the chemical nature of all the migrants is not known, the guidance recommends the use of solvents with different chemical characteristics such as polarity, aromaticity, etc. Both polar and nonpolar solvents should be used. Charged or very polar species such as heavy metals, catalyst complexes, and inorganic chemicals may also migrate from the polymers and would not be soluble in nonpolar solvents. Initial experiments should use a solvent of mixed polarity such as methylene dichloride. For highly crosslinked polymers, solvents that swell the polymer are desirable, as they would enable completion of the physicochemical characterization with a shorter extraction period.

The standardized solvent extraction techniques for biocompatibility assays were selected on the dual basis of simulating the conditions of clinical use of the product and choosing a solvent that itself would not adversely affect the assay model. The use of biocompatible solvents effectively sets a limit on the rate and amount of chemicals that will be extracted. Physicochemical characterization studies may demonstrate the total amount of an extractable substance exceeds the amount in a standardized extract preparation. In this case, investigations of the biological effects of the pure chemical may be desirable.

Detailed Description of Biocompatibility Procedures

This section provides a description of the methodology for the biocompatibility procedures. The selection of a biological model for in vitro or in vivo assays is based on the rationale and requirements for the investigation. Biocompatibility, safety, toxicity, and effectiveness studies are usually performed in animal models and/or species which have become generally accepted or historically selected based on considerations of availability, economic factors, anatomical features, physiological characteristics, biological responsiveness, ethical issues, and accumulated knowledge. In some cases, the particular strain of animal or cell is also relevant for evaluating the results of a bioassay because of unique biochemical pathways.

The process of standards development has followed the paradigm of comparing the responsiveness of a specific method or protocol for a selected set of materials or chemicals. The process may be done by a single investigator (an intra-laboratory study) or in cooperation with other investigators (inter-laboratory studies). Validation may be based on comparison with a defined benchmark such as correlation with another bioassay, mechanistic knowledge, or human data. For example, guinea pigs were found to be the most sensitive animal model for assessing delayed immune hypersensitivity. Similarly, rabbits were found to be the most sensitive animal species for detecting pyrogens in vivo. Rodents are used in single dose, repeated dose and lifetime studies because of the rationale for the assay, and secondary factors of availability, economic factors, and accumulated knowledge. These same considerations are important in selecting a nonrodent species for general toxicity assays. Rabbits are the species of choice for vascular irritation studies because of the large ear vein and its accessibility. Rabbits are also appropriate models for dermal irritation assays based on the similarity of their skin's responsiveness in comparison to that of human skin. Anatomical factors have a decisive role in the selection of animal models for oral, vaginal, and penile mucosal irritation assays.

In the case of efficacy testing of externally communicating or implanted medical devices, physical size, anatomy, and surgical technique are important constraints in combination with availability and ethical issues. Total blood volume affects which animals may be considered in efficacy testing of oxygenators, hemodialyzers, or apheresis devices. Anatomical and species differences in blood coagulation have a significant impact in selecting a large animal model for evaluating the efficacy of ventricular assist devices and total artificial hearts. Bovine species, for example, develop thrombi in peripheral tissues but not in the brain whereas in humans, brain strokes are the primary mode of failure (Didisheim, 1997). Surgical technique and therapeutic use of antibiotics and anticoagulants are especially relevant in efficacy testing of vascular access devices. National laws differ on the availability and use of primate species and human blood. A more comprehensive discussion of these variables may be obtained by searching the literature.

Cytotoxicity

Three in vitro cytotoxicity assays are described in ISO 10993 standard, Biological Evaluation of Medical devices—Part 5: Tests for Cytotoxicity: In Vitro Methods. The three primary methods are an extract test, a direct contact test, and an indirect contact test. These correspond to the methods established in the U.S. Pharmacopeia <87> Biological Reactivity, In vitro. The test samples are either a solid material or an extract prepared with either culture medium with or without serum, 0.9 % saline or other suitable solvent. Extraction time and temperature are those described above. Selection of the appropriate test is based on the nature of the sample to be evaluated, the potential site of use, and the nature of use. The direct and indirect assays are preferred for synthetic polymers that are likely to have water insoluble additives that may be extracted in a less polar solvent such as serum containing culture medium. Aqueous extracts are particularly useful for natural elastomers such as latex rubbers because natural elastomers generally contain water-soluble additives or reaction products.

The tests preferably use established adherent cell lines such as CCL1 (NCTC clone L-929), CCL 163 (Balb/3T3 clone A312), CCL 171 (MRC-5), CCL 75 (WI-38), CCL 81 (Vero), CCL 10 (BHK-21) or V-79 379A. The cell lines listed reflect the experiences of the task force involved in developing the standard. Cell lines, by definition, have dedifferentiated to some extent from the species and tissue of origin. Therefore, species distinctions may be relevant semantically but not necessarily from a biocompatibility perspective. Jarkelid et al (1997) compared the sensitivity of L-929 cells with five others that were used in the Multicentre Evaluation In Vitro Cytotoxicity Program. This interlaboratory trial evaluated the relevance and reliability of specific in vitro cytotoxicity tests as alternatives or supplements to animal tests. Using the uptake of a neutral red dye as a quantitative endpoint for determining the concentration of a test chemical that caused a 50% inhibition of cell growth (IC50), they found the correlation coefficient between the IC50 values from L-929 cells and the mean of five other cell models was 0.94 for 17 reference chemicals. The other cell models were HFL1, human fetal fibroblast cells; McCoy, human epithelial cells; MDBK, bovine kidney cells; rat hepatocytes; and Ascites Sarcoma BP8 cells. The ratio of the IC50 values from these cell models with L-929 cells varied between 1 and 9 for the nonvolatile chemicals and, in nine of the 17 tests, the L-929 cells were more sensitive than the cells used in the other methods.

Differences in the sensitivity of various adherent cell lines are often related to the cell density (i.e., the number of cells per unit of surface area). For example, Vero cells are much larger than the other cell lines, viz., sufficiently greater cell diameter such that the confluent, monolayer cell density is approximately half that of the L-929 cell line. This effectively increases the dose per Vero cell when compared to L-929 cells in monolayer cultures resulting in apparent, greater sensitivity of the Vero cells.

ISO 10993-5 requires three replicates rather than the two specified in the U.S. Pharmacopeia. The basis for increasing the number of replicates is to allow calculation of mean and standard deviation when quantitative endpoints are measured. However, the individual analyst should confirm that the tests are reproducible and adjust the number of replicates according to the statistical power of the assay and the probability of Type I or Type II errors.

The samples or extracts are added directly to culture vessels containing a monolayer of cells. Solid test samples are placed directly on a monolayer of cells (i.e., direct contact test), or on top of an agar gel overlay (i.e., indirect contact test). A fourth method, filter diffusion, requires growing the cells on a filter, inverting the cell-coated filter onto an agar layer (viz., apical side of the cells on the agar), and subsequent placement of the material or extract on the basal side of the cell-coated filter. The exposure period after addition of the test sample is 2 hours for the filter diffusion method, and 24 to 72 hours for the other methods. In the case of a colony-forming assay, which is required in Japan, the exposure period may be much longer because the time required for colony formation depends on the population doubling time of the particular cell line and the size of the colonies. Some cell lines may require a week of culturing to produce a sufficient number of colonies for evaluation.

A cytotoxic effect is evaluated by morphological means, measurements of cell damage, measurements of cell growth, or specific aspects of cellular metabolism. Table 4.2 gives the morphological ratings for cytotoxicity effects (US Pharmacopeia, 2000). A competent person, who is capable of making informed decisions based on the test data, makes an overall biocompatibility assessment. In general, a morphological rating of 2 or greater is considered a failure. The biological significance of the results of assays with quantitative measurements has not been standardized. Quantitative in vitro cytotoxicity assays that have good repeatability and reproducibility within a laboratory have not always been validated to ascertain their relationship with in vivo bioassays. Therefore, the interpretation may vary among testing laboratories.

The suitability of the cytotoxicity assays is often questioned whenever a material is associated with adverse effects. The appropriate, corrective action is to investigate the cause for the adverse outcome. Initial investigations will seek to confirm the reproducibility of sample preparation and conduct of the assay followed by inquiries on the physicochemical nature of the sample. Nonphysiological pH, extremes in osmolarity, surfactants, calcium chelating agents, antibiotics, or fixatives such as formaldehyde and glutaraldehyde are well-known sources for cytotoxic effects. A second action plan is to examine the dose-response relationship using serial, two-fold dilutions of an extract. This will provide information on the concentration of the toxic agent and its impact on the safety margin when compared with the clinical application. Additional materials characterization studies are described in Chapter 2.

Sensitization

Sensitization is the historical name for immunotoxicity. Immunotoxicity is any adverse effect mediated by changes in the immune system that is disproportionate to the toxicity manifested in other systems. The highly complex immune system has historically been subclassified into the cellular and humoral immune systems. The cellular immune system detects reactions between cells exemplified by the type IV delayed hypersensitivity reactions that occur in a localized tissue site. The humoral immune system detects circulating antibodies in the vascular system such as immunoglobulin E. This historical subdivision of the immune system is the foundation for the assays most frequently used to establish whether or not a medical device affects the immune system.

Immunotoxicity studies have traditionally focused on assessing delayed contact hypersensitivity (viz., cellular immunity) by the maximization or closed patch methods. Cellular immunity assays are effective in detecting low molecular weight, reactive molecules extracted from medical devices or their reactive metabolites which function as haptens and covalently bind to endogenous cells such as lymphocytes, macrophages and other antigen presenting cells. Humoral immunoassays detect antibodies that react with soluble antigens. Ethylene oxide is an example of an immunoreactive chemical found in medical devices (Rockel et al, 1986). Under appropriate conditions, ethylene oxide binds to serum albumin to form a potent antigen (Chapman et al, 1996). The potency of an antigen depends on persistent exposure to allow for recruitment and transformation of lymphocytes and clonal expansion of the antibody forming cells. That is, the immune potency of an antigen is related to differences in the rate of metabolism and elimination of an antigen at various anatomical sites. Exposure at a subcutaneous site which has limited metabolic capacity is more likely to induce an immune response (assuming the article is immunogenic) than exposure by the vascular route where the chemical may be rapidly metabolized.

Table 4.2. Reactivity grades for in vitro cytotoxicity assays*

Grade	Reactivity	Description of Reactivity Zone
		Agar diffusion and direct contact tests
0	None	No detectable zone around or under specimen
1	Slight	Some malformed or degenerated cells under specimen
2	Mild	Zone limited to area under specimen
3	Moderate	Zone extends 0.5 to 1.0 cm beyond specimen
4	Severe	Zone extends greater than 1.0 cm beyond specimen but does not involve entire dish
		Elution test
0	None	Discrete intracytoplasmic granules; no cell lysis
1	Slight	Not more than 20% of the cells are round, loosely attached, and without intracytoplasmic granules; occasional lysed cells are present
2	Mild	Not more than 50% of the cells are round and devoid of intracytoplasmic granules; extensive cell lysis and empty areas between cells
3	Moderate	Not more than 70% of the cell layers contain rounded cells and/or are lysed
4	Severe	Nearly complete destruction of the cell layers

*Reference: <87> Biological Reactivity Tests, In Vitro. US Pharmacopeia 2000; 24: 1831-1832.

Sensitization assays are described in ISO 10993 standard, Biological Evaluation of Medical devices—Part 10: Tests for Irritation and Delayed-type Hypersensitivity. The guinea pig maximization test (i.e., Magnusson and Kligman test) is used to determine if extracts of a test article cause delayed contact hypersensitivity, a reflection of immunogenic potential. During the induction phase of the test, animals are treated with pairs of intradermal injections and topical application of the (a) extract alone, (b) adjuvant alone and (c) extract-adjuvant mixture. The adjuvant enhances the number of lymphocytes that are recruited to the depot of the test and control substances. After one week, the extracts or controls are applied using filter paper and left in place for 48 hours. After a 2-week rest period, which allows replication and clonal expansion of the immunoreactive cells, the animals are challenged by topical application of the extract and covered with an occlusive patch for 24 hours. Skin reactions are rated for erythema and edema (Table 4.3) at 24, 48 and 72 hours after application of the extract. The material is considered to be a potential sensitizing agent if any animals give positive reactions. A similar protocol is followed in the Buehler assay for sensitization except that an adjuvant is not used.

Although it is not specified in the standard methods, a positive immune response may be confirmed by (a) testing the test animal's blood plasma in vitro to assess the presence of antibodies to the test agent and (b) extending the assay two weeks and rechallenging the test animals. An Oucterlony diffusion assay or immunoelectrophoresis method may be used to confirm or detect plasma antibodies against the test compound.

Langone (1998) published a framework for immunotoxicity evaluation of medical devices to assess the risks associated with use of a new medical device or material. This framework document recommends testing for five major immunological reactions that are found with medical device materials, i.e., hypersensitivity, inflammation, immunosuppression, immunostimulation, and autoimmunity. The extent of testing is dependent on the route and duration of body contact and whether the medical device is a plastic, polymer, metal, ceramic, or biological. Tables 4.4 and 4.5 list the specific immune responses associated with potential immunological effects and representative tests, indicators, and models for that assessment. Critical responses are those of primary importance as indications of immunotoxicity. Noncritical responses may also need to be evaluated for adequate safety, for example, when critical tests are positive or borderline. It is recommended that any clinical symptoms of immune system dysfunction are recorded and appropriate studies considered to understand the basis for these responses.

Irritation Assays

Irritation assays are described in ISO 10993 standard, Biological Evaluation of Medical devices—Part 10: Tests for Irritation and Delayed-type Hypersensitivity. The route of exposure subclassifies irritation tests, for example, skin, intracutaneous, eye and mucous membrane. These assays may be designed as single or repeated dose exposures. The detection limit of irritation assays often exceeds the systemic assays because the constituents are in immediate contact with target cells and there is less metabolism or dilution in the tissues or body fluids.

The intracutaneous irritation test in rabbits has been part of the basic safety evaluation battery of tests for medical devices for many years. It simulates the irritation which can occur in humans upon exposure of breached skin to a foreign irritating device or when the device is introduced subcutaneously. The method measures signs of inflammation as erythema, edema, ulceration and necrosis. Extracts are injected into the skin and the degree of irritation is assessed at 24, 48, and 72 hours. Skin reactions are evaluated using the scoring system in Table 4.3. A repeated-dose, dermal irritation assay is used for evaluating bandages, wound dressings, gloves, and other devices with repeated, longterm, skin contact. Eye irritation assays are particularly useful for evaluating contact lenses, and other medical devices that contact the ocular tissue. Mucosal membrane irritation assays are applicable to dental and personal hygiene devices. Intravascular irritation assays are applicable to externally communicating vascular devices such as catheters and cannulas.

Systemic Toxicity (Single and Repeated Dose Toxicity Including Pyrogenicity)

Single and repeated dose toxicity assays are designed to evaluate systemic responses following injection of extracts of test materials into laboratory animals. Systemic toxicity assays are listed in ISO 10993 standard, Biological Evaluation of Medical devices—Part 11: Tests for Systemic Toxicity. This standard covers tests for single (acute) and repeated dose toxicity and contains lists of recommendations of other standards for oral, dermal, inhalational, intravenous, and intraperitoneal routes of administration. It also cross-references the pyrogenicity tests described in pharmacopeias such as the European, Japanese and US Pharmacopeias.

Single dose systemic toxicity tests are designed to determine whether leachable materials induce mortality, body weight changes, or clinical signs of toxicity. The acute systemic toxicity test, which is described in the U.S. Pharmacopeia, is the most common assay for medical device biocompatibility testing. The test material is extracted in 9% saline, 5% ethanol in saline, vegetable oil, and polyethylene glycol 400. The former two extracts are injected intravenously and the latter two intraperitoneally into mice. The acute systemic toxicity assay is a maximum dose assay in that the dosage of 50 mL/kg bodyweight represents 5% of the total body weight and more than 50% of the blood volume. A bolus, intravenous dose of this size has immediate physiological effects on vascular volume and blood pressure. Thus, toxicological effects are readily evident if present, including the depression in activity from an intoxicating dose of ethanol from the 5% ethanol in saline extractant. The dosage for the Systemic Injection Test mimics that used in human therapy with hydration fluids such as physiological saline. Hydration therapy for a 60-kg human adult normally consists of 3,000 mL infused continuously

Table 4.3. Classification system for skin reaction*

Reaction	Numerical Grading
Erythema and eschar formation	
No erythema	0
Very slight erythema (barely perceptible)	1
Well-defined erythema	2
Moderate erythema	3
Severe erythema (beet-redness) to eschar formation	4
Edema formation	
No edema	0
Very slight edema (barely perceptible)	1
Well-defined edema (edges of area well-defined)	2
Moderate edema (raised approximately 1 mm)	3
Severe edema (raised more than 1 mm and extending beyond exposure area)	4

Reference: ISO 10993-10: Tests for irritation and delayed-type hypersensitivity.

Table 4.4. Classification of specific immune responses associated with potential immunological effects*

Immunological Effects	Histopathology	Humoral Response	Cellular Response T	NK	M	G	Host Response	Clinical Response
Delayed Hypersensitivity	NC	C	C	NA	NA	C	NA	C
Inflammation	C	NC	C	NA	C	C	C	C
Immunosuppression	NC	C	C	C	C	NA	NC	C
Immunostimulation	NC	C	C	NA	NC	NA	NC	C
Autoimmunity	C	C	C	NA	NA	NC	NC	C

Abbrev.: C, critical; NC, noncritical; NA, not applicable or not needed; T, T cells; NK, natural killer cells; M, macrophages; G, granulocytes (basophil, eosinophils and/or neutrophils).
*Reference: Langone JJ. Immunotoxicity testing guidance. US Food and Drug Administration, Center for Devices and Radiological Health, Office of Science and Technology, Rockville, MD. Draft document April 6, 1998.

over 24 hours [viz., 3000 mL/60 kg = 50 mL/kg bodyweight (bw)]. A reasonable safety margin for acute exposure was designed into the Systemic Injection Assay by increasing the infusion rate when compared to the clinical application. For example, a safety margin of 24 is achieved when the 24-hour clinical rate is reduced to the equivalent of a 60-minute infusion rate. That is, 3000 mL/60 kg bw/24 hours = 0.034 mL/kg/min is reduced to 3000 mL/60 kg bw/hr = 50 mL/kg bw/hr or 0.83 mL/kg bw/min. Increasing the infusion rate (i.e., decreasing the time for infusion) beyond a nominal rate of 1 mL/min results in significant, increased risk of cardiovascular failure from the rapid expansion of vascular volume. The mice are observed daily for 72 hours. In some cases, a bodyweight loss or failure to gain weight may be the only evidence of an adverse effect following a single dose of a test solution.

Table 4.5. Representative tests, indicators, and models for the evaluation of immune responses*

Immune Response	Functional Assays	Phenotyping	Soluble Mediators	Other
Histopathology	Not applicable	Cell surface markers	Not applicable	Morphology
Humoral Response	Immunoassays for antibody response to antigen plus adjuvant, plaque-forming cells, lymphocyte proliferation, antibody-dependent cell-mediated cytotoxicity, passive cutaneous anaphylaxis, direct anaphylaxis	Cell surface markers	Complement (including C3a and C5a anaphylatoxins), immune complexes	
Cellular Response:				
T Cells	Guinea pig maximization test, mouse local lymph node assay, mouse ear swelling test, lymphocyte proliferation, mixed lymphocyte reaction	Cell surface markers (helper and cytotoxic T cells)	Cytokine patterns indicative of T cell subset (e.g., Th 1 and Th 2)	
Natural Killer Cells	Tumor cytotoxicity	Cell surface markers	Not applicable	
Macrophages	Antigen presentation, phagocytosis	MHC markers	Cytokines (IL-1, TNF-alpha, IL-6, TGF-beta)	
Granulocytes†	Phagocytosis, degranulation	Not applicable	Chemokines, bioactive amines Inflammatory cytokines, enzymes	Cytochemistry
Host Resistance	Resistance to bacteria, viruses, and tumors	Not applicable	Not applicable	
Clinical Symptoms	Not applicable	Not applicable	Not applicable Not applicable	Allergy, skin rash, urticaria, edema, lymphadenopathy

Abbrev.: IL, interleukin; MHC, major histocompatibility complex; TGF, tumor growth factor; TNF, tumor necrosis factor.
†Basophils, eosinophils and/or neutrophils.
*Reference: Langone JJ. Immunotoxicity testing guidance. US Food and Drug Administration, Center for Devices and Radiological Health, Office of Science and Technology, Rockville, MD. Draft document April 6, 1998.

The outcome of the systemic toxicity assays may be affected by factors other than intrinsic toxicity of the test sample. False positive responses may result, for example, from the viscosity of extracts from hydrocolloid wound dressings, excess particulate, or nonphysiological pH. The amount of extractable constituents from insoluble medical devices also may not reach sufficient concentration levels in the vehicle to cause acute effects. This is very often the case with aqueous vehicles, which extract limited amounts of water insoluble chemicals.

Repeated dose and chronic toxicity tests are performed in rodent and nonrodent species. Table 4.6 presents the number of animals recommended for repeated dose and chronic toxicity tests. This table was derived from guidelines and requirements published by the U.S. FDA and other national health agencies. It is evident that the number of animals increases with the length of the study. ISO 10993 standards, Biological Evaluation of Medical devices—Part 6: Tests for Local Effects after Implantation and Part 11: Tests for Systemic Toxicity provide very limited guidance on the conduct of repeated and chronic dose testing. ISO 10993—Part 6 has the narrow focus of only evaluating subcutaneous muscle and bone implantation sites after 1, 4, 12, 26, 52, and 78 weeks in most species and additional observations at 3, 9, and 104 weeks in selected species. ISO 10993—Part 11 merely provides references to other standards which were designed for noninvasive repeated dose toxicity studies such as an oral feeding study, inhalation exposure, and repeated skin applications. In this author's opinion, the study designs that will be most appropriate for medical devices are most likely to include variables named in existing standards along with those unique concerns for assessing the safety and efficacy of a given medical device. These concepts are briefly discussed herein.

The biocompatibility for repeated exposure to surface-contacting devices is assessed by daily exposure of the test animal to the device or material. Bandages, wound dressings, and surgical gowns, for example, would be applied to the intact skin on a daily basis. Standard exposure periods are 1, 2, and 4 weeks with exceptional studies of greater duration. Generally, the sample is covered with an impermeable barrier to enhance hydration from perspiration and the probability of skin permeation of any extractable chemicals. The test and control sites are evaluated daily for erythema and edema (see Table 4.3) and at the termination of the study. Histopathological examination of the test and control sites permits distinguishing an inflammatory reaction from an immune reaction. A more thorough protocol would evaluate blood biochemistry and histopathology of various organs and tissues because the design of the study includes evaluation of the effects of absorbed chemicals rather than only a localized skin reaction.

Repeated dose safety testing of externally communicating devices often involves testing an extract of the device in a physiologically compatible solvent. For example, extracts from a hemodialiyzer might be tested by repeated intravenous injection. The duration of an intravenous study with consecutive, daily dosing in a rodent model depends on expertise in dosing the animals without causing excessive injury to the veins or complications from infections. The use of implanted catheters for vein access potentially offers the advantage of extending the study duration but may cause complications from clotting and infection around the catheter. Thus, to obtain high quality data in a rodent model, a 28-day repeated dose study with direct intravenous injections may be the best design. Longer, repeated dose studies are highly dependent on the technical skills of the investigator. Daily dosing is recommended in order to increase the blood concentration of the extracted chemicals and because the data are used to extrapolate safety for a human population whose deficient kidney function results in impaired elimination of waste. The parameters for the preparation of the hemodialyzer extracts will need to rationalize how to obtain an extract which can be infused in a reasonable dose volume (less than 40 mL/kg bodyweight) and rate of administration while also providing a margin of safety in comparison to the predicted patient dose of extractable chemicals. Observations and measurements conducted during the pretreatment and treatment phases include ophthalmic examinations, body weights, clinical observations, and, where possible, pretreatment urinalysis and

Table 4.6. Numbers of animals per dosage group in nonacute toxicity studies

Study Duration	**Rodents (per sex)**	**Nonrodents (per sex)**
2-4 weeks	5	3
13 weeks	20[1]	6
26 weeks	30	8
1 year	50	10
Carcinogenicity bioassays	60[2]	Applies only to contraceptives

[1] Starting with 13-week studies, one should consider adding animals (particularly to the high dose) to allow evaluation of reversal of effects.
[2] In recent years, there have been decreasing levels of survival in rats on 2-year studies. What is required is that at least 20-50 animals/sex/group survive at the end of the study. Accordingly, practice is beginning to use 70 to 75 animals per sex, per group.

blood tests. At the termination of the study, biological samples are evaluated for hematological and biochemical parameters, and urinalyses. Each animal is autopsied and the tissues examined for pathological changes. Table 4.7 contains a list of the assays and tissues that are included in single and repeated dose toxicology studies to comply with internationally harmonized practices for quality studies and meet international regulatory requirements.

Many of the design considerations for the repeated dose studies would be included in longterm implantation studies. A vascular implantation study would incorporate additional measurements of hemocompatibility as listed in Table 4.8 and 4.9. Particulate formation at the sight of the implant and migration via the vascular or lymphatic systems to distal tissues also may occur, especially if the device was implanted in vascular tissue, made from a flexible polymer or gel, or implanted in an articulating joint such as the hip or knee. In this event, histopathology studies for particulate around the implant and in distal tissues such as lung, liver, spleen and kidneys are relevant for establishing safety.

Pyrogenicity

The cell wall of gram-negative bacteria contains endotoxins, which are lipophilic molecules that cause febrile reactions in humans and animals. In vitro and in vivo tests have been developed to determine the presence of endotoxins. The bacterial endotoxins test, which is also known as the *Limulus* amoebocyte lysate (LAL) test, measures the concentration of endotoxins using either a turbidimetric or colorimetric endpoint (USP monograph <85> Bacterial Endotoxins Test). The LAL endotoxin limit for transfusion and infusion assemblies is not to exceed 0.5 USP Endotoxin Units (EU) per mL when 40 mL of water is passed through each of ten assemblies at a flow rate of 10 mL per minute and a temperature between 37 and 40°C (USP monograph <161> Transfusion and Infusion Assemblies). The LAL endotoxin limit for implanted medical devices is 0.5 EU per mL when 3 to 10 sterile implants are soaked in 400 mL of water for 40 to 60 minutes at a temperature between 37 and 40°C. Medical devices in contact with cerebrospinal fluid have an LAL endotoxin limit of less than 0.06 EU. There are cases when a pyrogenic effect would not be detected with the bacterial endotoxins test, for example, devices based on biological materials. In such circumstances, the rabbit pyrogenicity test should be used.

The rabbit pyrogen test is designed to limit the risks of febrile reactions to an acceptable level (USP monograph <151> Pyrogen Test). The test involves measuring the rise in temperature of rabbits over a 3-hour interval following the intravenous injection of a test solution. The sample passes the test if no rabbit shows an individual rise in temperature of 0.5°C or more above its respective control temperature.

Genotoxicity

Genotoxicity assays are described in ISO 10993 standard, Biological Evaluation of Medical devices—Part 3: Tests for Genotoxicity, Carcinogenicity and Reproductive toxicity. The standard recommends in vitro testing in two mammalian cell systems, and one nonmammalian system using assays for effects on deoxynucleic acid (DNA), gene mutations, and chromosomal aberrations. Testing would not be required if the devices are made from materials known to show no genotoxicity or if all components in extracts of the device can be identified by suitable analytical methods and have been shown to have no genetic effects. Assays may be performed with extracts of the intact or dissolved material. Physiological saline and dimethyl sulfoxide are recommended as suitable extractant media. The extracts are prepared at 37°C for a minimum of 24 hours using the highest possible surface area per volume of extractant in closed containers with minimum headspace. The latter requirement is to minimize the loss of the volatile constituents. The specific methods are those published by the Organization of Economic Cooperation and Development (Table 4.10). More recently, the International Conference on Harmonization of testing for pharmaceutical products has recommended three assays as the preferred genotoxicity assays (see www.pharmweb.net/pwmirror/pw9/ifpma/ich1.html). This guidance recommends in vitro bacterial assays using selected *Salmonella typhimurium* or *Escherichia coli* strains, an in vivo rodent bone marrow assay, and a rodent bone marrow micronucleus assay. It is predicted that the International Conference on Harmonization recommendations will predominate in the future.

The *Salmonella typhimurium* or Ames assay is historically the most widely employed genotoxicity test for screening potential carcinogens. It is one of the few established short-term tests in which large numbers of both carcinogens and noncarcinogens, representing a wide variety of chemical classes, have been tested using a defined protocol. This very sensitive assay determines the potential of a test material to induce the genetic mutation of histidine reversion using 5 strains of *Salmonella typhimurium* (viz., TA 98, TA 100, TA 1535, TA 1537, and TA 102) that are extremely sensitive to DNA-damaging agents in the presence or absence of mammalian enzymes. *Escherichia coli* strains WP2 *uvr*A or *uvr*A (pKM101) may be substituted for *S. typhimurium* TA102. This assay is considered a reliable predictor in that a positive response in the *Salmonella* mutagenicity assay can be used to infer carcinogenicity in rodents (Tennant et al 1987).

The bacterial reverse mutation tests use amino-acid requiring strains of *Salmonella typhimurium* and *Escherichia coli* to detect point mutations, which involve substitution, addition or deletion of one or a few DNA base pairs. Strains TA98, TA100, TA 1535, and TA 1537 detect changes at guanosine-cytosine sites within target genes whereas TA102 detects modifications of the adenine-thymine base pairs. The principle of the bacterial reverse mutation test is that it detects mutations that functionally reverse mutations present in the test strains and restore the capability to synthesize an essential amino acid. The revertant cells are detected by their ability to grow in the absence of the amino acid required by the parent test strain.

The test directly measures DNA mutations of a type that is associated with adverse affects. Point mutations are the cause of many human genetic diseases and there is substantial evidence that point mutations in oncogenes and tumor suppressor genes of somatic cells are involved in tumor formation in humans and experimental animals. Many of the test strains have several features that make them more sensitive for the detection of mutations including responsive

Table 4.7. Clinical and anatomical pathology measurements for nonclinical studies

Hematology	
Red blood cell count	Differential blood cell count
Hemoglobin	Nucleated red blood cell count
Plasma hemoglobin	Corrected white blood cell count
Hematocrit	Segmented neutrophil count
Mean corpuscular volume	Band neutrophil count
Mean corpuscular hemoglobin	Lymphocyte count
Mean corpuscular hemoglobin concentration	Monocyte count
Platelet count	Eosinophil count
White blood cell count	Basophil count
Blood cell morphology	
Clinical Chemistry	
Glucose	Aspartate aminotransferase
Urea nitrogen	Alanine aminotransferase
Creatinine	Gamma-glutamyl transferase
Total protein	Calcium
Albumin	Inorganic phosphorus
Globulin	Sodium
Total bilirubin	Potassium
Cholesterol	Chloride
Triglycerides	
Histopathology	
Adrenals	Nasal cavity
Aorta	Ovaries
Brain	Pancreas
Cecum	Pituitary
Colon	Prostate
Duodenum	Rectum
Epididymis	Salivary gland (sumaxillary)
Esophagus	Sciatic nerve
Eyes	Seminal vesicles
Femur with bone marrow	Skin
(articular surface of the distal end)	Spinal cord (cervical, mid-thoracic, and lumbar)
Gallbladder	Spleen
Heart	Sternum with bone marrow
Ileum	Stomach
Jejunum	Testes
Kidneys	Treatment site
Lacrimal gland (exorbital)	Thymus
Lesions	Thyroids with parathyroid
Liver	Tongue
Lungs	Trachea
Lymph node (mesenteric and submaxillary)	Urinary bladder
Mammary gland (females only)	Uterus
Muscle (thigh)	Vagina

Table 4.8. Required hemocompatibility tests for external communicating and implanted devices*

Device Category	Test Category	Method
External communicating	Thrombosis	Light microscopy of adhered platelets, leucocytes, aggregates, erythrocytes, fibrin, etc.
Blood path, indirect	Coagulation	Partial thromboplastin time
	Platelets	Platelet count
	Hematology	Leucocyte and differential; hemolysis (plasma hemoglobin)
	Immunology	Complement activation (C3a, C5a, TCC, Bb, iC3b, C4d, SC5B-9)
External communicating circulating blood	Thrombosis	Percent occlusion; flow reduction; thrombus mass; light microscopy; pressure drop across device
	Coagulation	Partial thromboplastin time
	Platelets	Platelet count; platelet aggregation, template bleeding time
	Hematology	Leucocyte and differential; hemolysis (plasma hemoglobin)
	Immunology	Complement activation (C3a, C5a, TCC, Bb, iC3b, C4d, SC5B-9)
Implanted devices	Thrombosis	Percent occlusion; flow reduction; autopsy of device (gross and microscopic); autopsy of distal organs (gross and microscopic)
	Coagulation	Partial thromboplastin time, prothrombin time, thrombin time, plasma fibrinogen, fibrin degradation products
	Platelets	Platelet count; platelet aggregation
	Hematology	Leucocyte and differential; hemolysis (plasma hemoglobin)
	Immunology	Complement activation (C3a, C5a, TCC, Bb, iC3b, C4d, SC5B-9)

Abbreviations: Bb, product of alternate pathway of complement activation; C3a, complement split product from C3; C4d, product of classical pathway of complement activation; C5a, complement split product from C5; iC3b, product of central C complement activation; SC5B-9, product of terminal pathway of complement activation; TCC, terminal complement complex.
Reference: ISO 10993-4: Selection of tests for interactions with blood.

DNA sequences at the reversion sites, increased cell permeability to large molecules, and elimination of DNA repair systems or enhancement of error-prone DNA repair processes. The specificity of the test strains can provide some useful information on the types of mutations that are induced by genotoxic agents.

The bacterial reverse mutation test utilizes prokaryotic cells (i.e., lacking a nucleus), which differ from mammalian cells in such factors as uptake, metabolism, chromosome structure, and DNA repair processes. Tests conducted in vitro generally require the use of an exogenous source of metabolic activation. The tests provide indirect rather than direct information on mutagenic and carcinogenic potency in mammals because the in vitro metabolic activation systems used in the tests cannot mimic entirely the mammalian in vivo conditions.

Table 4.9. Optional hemocompatibility tests for external communicating and implanted devices

Device Category	Test Category	Method
External communicating or Implanted devices	Thrombosis	Scanning electron microscopy; angiography
	Coagulation	Specific coagulation assays as fibrinopeptide A, D-dimer, prothrombin activation fragment 1+2, thrombin-antithrombin complex.
	Platelets	Platelet factor 4, beta-thromboglobulin, thromboxane B2, platelet survival, gamma imaging of radiolabelled platelets
	Hematology	Reticulocyte count, activation-specific release products of peripheral blood cells (i.e., granulocytes)
	Immunology	Interleukin-1 and other cytokines, messenger-RNA for specific cytokines

Reference: ISO 10993-4: Selection of tests for interactions with blood.

Tests measuring chromosomal aberration in nucleated bone marrow cells in rodents can detect a wide spectrum of changes in chromosomal integrity. Breakage of one or more chromatids or chromosomes can result in micronucleus formation or chromosomal aberrations. These are detected either by measurement of micronucleated polychromatic erythrocytes in bone marrow cells or analysis of chromosomal aberrations. The measurement of micronucleated, immature (e.g., polychromatic) erythrocytes in peripheral blood is an acceptable alternative in the mouse, or other species in which the inability of the spleen to remove micronucleated erythrocytes has been demonstrated. The in vivo tests have the advantage of taking into account absorption, distribution, and excretion, processes that are not functional in in vitro tests. The significance of in vivo results in genotoxicity test strategies is directly related to the demonstration of adequate exposure of the target tissue to the test compound. If adequate exposure cannot be achieved, then conventional in vivo genotoxicity tests may have limited value.

Implantation

Implantation assays examine the in vivo tissue response to the test material implanted in an appropriate tissue for periods of 1 week and extending up to the animals' lifetime. Tissue specimens, explanted at intervals, are evaluated by macroscopic and microscopic pathology for the nature and degree of host tissue and inflammatory responses around the implant site.

Different biomaterials implanted in the body stimulate the proliferation of fibrous tissue in which fibroblasts surround the implant as early as seven days. The amount of fibrous tissue proliferation varies with the nature of the material, surface treatment, tissue site, and method of implantation. Excessive tissue response may be perceived as tissue incompatibility. Selection of materials to control the repopulating of a wound by a preferred tissue type has been given the metaphor of guided tissue regeneration (Ashammakhi, 1996).

Implantation assays are described in ISO 10993 standard, Biological Evaluation of Medical devices—Part 6: Tests for Local Effects after Implantation. The document contains a description of common provisions and more detailed descriptions of methods for implantation

Table 4.10. OECD guidelines for testing of chemicals—genotoxicity assays

Exposure	Identifier	Title
In vitro	471	Genetic Toxicology: *Salmonella typhimurium,* Reverse Mutation Assay.
	472	Genetic Toxicology: *Escherichia Coli,* Reverse Mutation Assay.
	473	Genetic Toxicology: In vitro Mammalian Cytogenic Test.
	476	Genetic Toxicology: Mammalian Cell Gene Mutation Test.
	479	Genetic Toxicology: In vitro sister chromatid Exchange Assay in Mammalian Cells.
	480	Genetic Toxicology: *Saccharomyces cereviside,* Gene Mutation Assay.
	481	Genetic Toxicology: *Saccharomyces cereviside,* Mitotic Recombination Assay.
	482	Genetic Toxicology: DNA Damage and Repair/Unscheduled DNA Synthesis in Mammalian Cells in vitro.
In vivo	474	Genetic Toxicology: Micronucleus Test.
	475	Genetic Toxicology: In vivo Mammalian Bone Marrow Cytogentic Test—Chromosomal Analysis.
	478	Genetic Toxicology: Rodent Dominant Lethal Test.
	483	Genetic Toxicology: Mammalian Germ-cell Cytogentic Assay.
	484	Genetic Toxicology: Mouse Spot Test.
	485	Genetic Toxicology: Mouse Heritable Translocation Assay.

Reference: www.oecd.org

in subcutaneous tissue, muscle, and bone. The local effects are evaluated by a comparison of the tissue response caused by a test specimen to that caused by materials used in medical devices whose clinical acceptability has been established and/or to standard reference materials. The duration of the tests are short-term (described as up to 12 weeks) and chronic (greater than 12 weeks implantation). Solid implants or nonsolid materials (liquids, pastes, and particulate) are included in the document. The nonsolid specimens are contained in tubes of polyethylene, polypropylene, or polytetrafluoroethylene. All specimens are processed, cleaned, and sterilized by the method intended for the final product. The size and shape of the test and control implants is determined by the investigator in consideration of the physical limitations of the animal species and implantation site. Table 4.11 lists the recommended specimen dimensions for implantation into subcutaneous tissue. For rabbit paravertebral muscles, implants of a width of 1-3 mm diameter and a length of approximately 10-mm are specified. For bone implantation, cylindrical specimens of 2 by 6-mm diameter are recommended for rabbits whereas specimens of 4 by 12-mm diameter are recommended for dogs, sheep, and goats. The size for orthopedic screw-type implants is 2-4.5 mm diameter for rabbits, dogs, sheep, goats, and pigs. A third dimension that should be considered is the relative size difference between the host and the material. That is, how much material surface area is the host being exposed to? The material surface area to body weight ratio may become a significant factor for porous materials and devices of repeated short-term applications (for example, hemodialysis and hemofiltration products).

The ISO standard provides abbreviated directions for implantation by hypodermic needle, trocar, and surgical techniques. All surgical techniques require local or general anesthesia to minimize trauma and provide for humane care of the animals. The investigator determines the test species and duration of implantation. Mice, rats, guinea pigs, and rabbits are recommended for implantation periods of 12 weeks or less in subcutaneous tissue and muscle. Rats, guinea

Table 4.11. Test specimens for subcutaneous implantation

Material Form	Subcutaneous Tissue
Sheet material	10-12 mm diameter by 0.3-1 mm thick
Bulk Materials	1.5 mm diameter by 5 mm length
Grooved specimens	4 mm diameter by 7 mm length
Nonsolid specimens	1.5 mm diameter by 5-mm length tubes

Reference: ISO 10993-6 Tests for Local Effects after Implantation.

pigs, rabbits, dogs, sheep, goats, and pigs are recommended for long-term implantation in subcutaneous tissue, muscle, and bone. Table 4.12 lists the number of test and control implantation specimens by tissue site. Although biostatistical analysis has not been a common concern in the past for nonclinical studies, it is becoming an issue of greater interest. Consequently, the number of animals used in a study and the test protocol should be evaluated to determine whether the biostatistical concerns are met.

At the termination of the implantation period, the animals are euthanized, and the biological response is evaluated by macroscopic and histological methods. The control and test implants and surrounding tissue are compared at equivalent locations relative to each implant so that the effect of relative motion between the tissue and implant is at a minimum. Embedding of the intact tissue envelope with the implant in situ in hard plastic is preferred for the assessment of the implant-tissue interface. Biological parameters to be assessed include: a) extent of fibrosis, fibrous capsule and inflammation; b) degeneration as determined by changes in tissue morphology; c) number and distribution of inflammatory cells such as polymorphonuclear leucocytes, lymphocytes, plasma cells, eosinophils, macrophages and multinucleated cells as a function of distance from the material-tissue interface; d) presence of necrosis as determined by nuclear debris and/or capillary wall breakdown; e) other parameters such as material debris, fatty infiltration, granuloma, and the quality and quantity of tissue ingrowth into porous implant materials.

Notably, the standard does not mention assessment of effects in distal tissues, hematology, clinical biochemistry, bodyweight, or other parameters commonly evaluated in toxicity studies of comparable duration. These measures would be included in the evaluation of a resorbable material, cardiovascular devices, and studies intended to meet the requirements of a carcinogenicity bioassay.

Hemocompatibility

Hemocompatibility assays are described in ISO 10993 standard, Biological Evaluation of Medical devices—Part 4: Selection of Tests for Interactions with Blood. This document is a guide for evaluating the interaction of medical devices with blood and was derived from a report prepared by the National Heart, Lung, and Blood Institute (1985). The standard lists recommended test methods (Tables 4.8 and 4.9) for medical devices externally communicating with the blood path, those communicating with circulating blood, and devices implanted in the cardiovascular system. Examples of externally communicating devices are cannulae, extension sets, devices for the collection of blood, and devices for the storage of blood and blood products. Examples of devices communicating with circulating blood are cardiopulmonary bypass devices, extracorporeal membrane oxygenators, hemodialysis equipment, apheresis equipment, devices for absorption of specific substances from blood, percutaneous circulatory support systems, and temporary pacemaker electrodes. Examples of devices implanted in the

Table 4.12. Test animals and implant sites

Tissue	No.Animals	No.Test Implants	No. Controls
Subcutaneous	At least 3 mice, rats, guinea pigs, or rabbits	10	10
Muscle	At least 3 of each specie	4/rabbit; total of 8 specimens for larger species	4/rabbit; total of 8 specimens for larger species
Bone	At least 4 rabbits or 2 dogs, sheep, goats, or pigs	3/rabbit; 6 implants in other species	3/rabbit; 6 implants in larger species

Reference: ISO 10993-6 Tests for Local Effects after Implantation.

cardiovascular system are heart valves, vascular grafts, circulatory support devices, blood filters, stents, arteriovenous shunts, blood monitors, pacemaker electrodes, and artificial lungs. It is recommended that devices whose intended use is ex vivo (external communicating) be tested in ex vivo assays and that implanted devices be tested in an animal model under conditions simulating clinical use. Devices that come into very brief contact with circulating blood (e.g., lancets, hypodermic needles, and capillary tubes) generally do not require blood/device interaction testing.

The predictability of the hemocompatibility tests are dependent on simulating the geometry and conditions of contact of the device with blood during clinical applications, including selective use of anticoagulants if appropriate. The document recommends the use of human blood in the assays where possible because of species differences in reactivity. However, it also recognizes that tests in animals or with animal blood may be necessary for various reasons. That is, preliminary tests in animals or with blood from animals are useful in identifying materials or design factors associated with lower hemocompatibility performance characteristics than a marketed product. Nonhuman primates such as baboons bear a close similarity to the human in hematologic values, blood coagulation mechanisms, and cardiovascular system. The dog is also a commonly used species, however, device-related thrombosis in the dog tends to occur more readily than in the human. The pig is generally regarded as a suitable animal model because of its hematologic and cardiovascular similarities to the human. Differences in design, changes in surface or bulk chemical composition of materials, and changes in texture, porosity, or other properties at the blood/material interface may have significant effects on the clinical function of a medical device.

Hemocompatibility testing methods are broadly categorized by the primary process or system being measured: thrombosis, coagulation, platelets and platelet functions, hematology, and immunology. The recommended measurements by hemocompatibility and device exposure category are listed in Table 4.8. Optional tests for hemocompatibility are listed in Table 4.9. The optional tests generally require more specialized equipment or methods that are species specific. For devices with limited blood exposure (< 24 hours), important measurements are related to the extent of variation of hematologic, hemodynamic and performance variables, gross thrombus formation, and thromboembolism. With prolonged or repeated exposure, or permanent contact (> 24 hours), emphasis is placed on serial measurement techniques that may yield information regarding the time course of thrombosis and thromboembolism, the consumption of circulating blood components, the development of intimal hyperplasia, and infection. Hemolysis is important for either exposure scenario. The consequences of the interaction of artificial surfaces with blood may range from gross thrombosis and embolization to subtle effects such as accelerated consumption of hemostatic elements, which may be compensated or lead to depletion of platelets or plasma coagulation factors. Activated blood coagulation and interactions between platelets, leucocytes, and complement may affect disturbances of kidney function and pulmonary function. The key role of platelets is in preventing bleeding. Platelet adhesion, platelet aggregation, platelet sequestration, or blood coagulation on materials or devices may cause a significant drop in the platelet count of blood exposed to a device. Leucocytes have an important role in immunocompetence. A reduced leukocyte count may signal leukocyte activation, aggregation, and removal from the circulation. An increased leukocyte count or a shift in the differential distribution of leukocyte subtypes (i.e., granulocytes, lymphocytes, and monocytes) may indicate a bacterial infection. The release of cytokines from leucocytes plays a major role in regulating the inflammatory response by controlling the growth of fibroblasts, smooth muscle cells, and endothelial cells.

The annexes of ISO 10993-4 provide an overview of the hemocompatibility assays, their relevance to medical device evaluation, and assays particularly suited to specific devices. The hemolysis assay, details of which are provided in the annex, determines the degree of cellular lysis following incubation of the test materials with isolated red blood cells under either static or dynamic conditions. The specific methods for other hemocompatibility tests are described in textbooks on hematology and clinical pathology. The interested reader is invited to consult these for a detailed discussion of methodology.

Application of the variety of hemocompatibility tests have been published by Rao and Sharms (1997). Chitosan was evaluated as a hemostatic agent for use in vascular grafts to reduce leakage following implantation. For this application, blood coagulation is a desirable property. Thus, coagulation, hemagglutination, and platelet adhesion tests were essential for demonstrating efficacy.

Chronic Toxicity and Carcinogenicity

Chronic systemic toxicity testing of medical devices is described in ISO 10993 standard, Biological Evaluation of Medical devices—Part 11: Tests for Systemic Toxicity. Where appropriate, chronic toxicity tests are often incorporated into a carcinogenicity bioassay.

Carcinogenicity assays are described in ISO 10993 standard, Biological Evaluation of Medical devices—Part 3: Tests for Genotoxicity, Carcinogenicity and Reproductive toxicity. Carcinogenicity assays are recommended for (a) resorbable materials and devices, unless there are significant and adequate data on human use or exposure; (b) materials and devices where positive results have been obtained in genetic toxicity testing on mammalian cells; and (c) materials and devices introduced in the body and/or its cavities with a permanent or cumulative contact of 30 days or longer, except when significant and adequate human-use history is available. The preferred route of exposure is implantation using two dose levels, i.e., the maximum implantable dose and a fraction thereof. The maximum implantable dose, a multiple of the worst case human exposure, should be expressed in device weight per kilogram of bodyweight. Carcinogenicity assays are normally performed in rodent species, starting at 6-8 weeks of age and continuing for the lifetime of the species, which is approximately 2 years. However, if there are a significant number of animal deaths, the assay should be terminated when there are 20-30 survivors per group. A minimum of 50 animals per test or control group is recommended to identify a difference of 2 animals with test related tumors [viz., (2/50) x 100 = 4%]. In recent years, the usual practice is to increase the number of animals per group to allow for interim sacrifices and to ensure adequate survival at the end of 2 years. Additional details on the conduct of tests for carcinogenicity and combined chronic toxicity and carcinogenicity studies are given in the OECD guidelines 451 and 453, respectively.

Carcinogenicity bioassays of solid materials in rodent species have been a subject of great concern because the data have not been predictive of human experience with the same materials. This phenomenon in experimental animals is known as solid state or foreign body carcinogenesis. It has been well-known for over 50 years that many materials independent of their chemical composition and dependent on their size, shape, surface characteristics, and duration of implantation will result in a high incidence of neoplasms in rats, mice, and hamsters. Guinea pigs and chickens, on the other hand, are resistant, and dogs appear to have an intermediate sensitivity. The foreign body neoplasms originate from the fibrous reaction surrounding the implant. Brand et al (1967) have shown that cell clones, apparently originating from the microvasculature, occur in the outer fibrous capsule reaction of mice as early as 4 weeks post-implantation. These cell clones are destined to become foreign body neoplasms. Before the neoplasms can occur, a series of key events is necessary. These include: (1) cellular proliferation and infiltration during the acute, foreign body reaction; (2) fibrosis of the tissue capsule around the foreign body; (3) quiescence of the tissue reaction (dormancy and inactivity of the foreign body attached macrophages); and (4) the availability of a foreign body surface with clonal preneoplastic cells. Neoplastic autonomy is reached when the clonal cells attach to the foreign body surface. This occurs approximately 6 to 7 months post-implantation. Based on the finding that a portion of the early 11 week capsule when explanted into genetically related animals would not form a neoplasm, Brand et al (1967) concluded there was no indication that the initial acquisition of neoplastic potential or the determination of specific tumor characteristic was based on direct physical or chemical contact between these cells and the foreign body.

Reproductive and Developmental Toxicity

Reproductive and developmental toxicity assays are described briefly in ISO 10993 standard, Biological Evaluation of Medical devices—Part 3: Tests for Genotoxicity, Carcinogenicity and Reproductive toxicity. These tests are recommended for intrauterine and contraceptive devices, longterm contact devices likely to come into direct contact with reproductive tissues or the embryo/fetus, and resorbable materials and devices that are used in women of childbearing age. Reproductive testing is not necessary if there are adequate data from absorption, metabolism, distribution, and reproductive effects of all major components identified in extracts of the device. The preferred route of exposure is implantation. Two dose levels, the maximum implantable dose and fraction thereof, are recommended. The maximum implantable dose, a multiple of the worst case human exposure, should be expressed as weight per kilogram of bodyweight. Additional details on the conduct of tests for teratogenicity and a one-generation reproduction toxicity study are given in the OECD guidelines 414 and 415, respectively.

Biodegradation

Biodegradation assays are described in ISO 10993 standard, Biological Evaluation of Medical devices—Part 9: Degradation of Materials Related to Biological Testing. Detailed, standard methods for degradation studies are given in parts 13, 14, and 15 of ISO 10993 for polymers, ceramics, and metals, respectively (see Chapter 2, Table 2.2). The term biodegradation is defined as an alteration of the biomaterial or medical device involving loss of integrity or performance in a physiological or simulated environment. Part 9 describes techniques and methods for in vitro degradation tests and techniques for identification and quantification of in vivo degradation products from medical implants. The report covers polymers, ceramics, carbons (pyrolytic carbons, graphites, and glassy or polymeric carbons), composites, metals, and alloys as well as coatings for these.

The human body is an aggressive environment for most types of materials or medical devices. Materials exposed to this environment undergo change as a result of chemical, physical, mechanical, and biological interactions of varying complexity and ultimately changing the properties and functionality of the medical devices. Ceramic materials, metals, and alloys undergo corrosion reactions through ion exchange and dissolution along with mechanical, cellular, and enzymatic degradation. The mechanisms of biodegration of polymers are attributed to surface erosion, mechanical stress cracking, phagocyte oxidants, oxidative and hydrolytic enzymes, or other chemical hydrolysis. The complexity of biodegradation is exemplified in the studies of Maurin et al (1997) who examined the in vivo degradation of a polyurethane powder in the peritoneal cavity of mice. Histological observations and morphological measurements of the deformation of the particles showed an initial swelling followed by mechanical stress cracking and thinning. These fragments were rapidly exposed to natural, peritoneal exudates responsible for enzymatic degradation. Enzymatic degradation was aided by the presence of cells in the fissures of the material. Additionally, cytokines released by the phagocytic cells may have modulated the cellular effects on degradation (Benahmed et al, 1997). In vitro studies have complemented the animal studies and support the role of oxidative and hydrolytic enzymes in combination with mechanical stresses.

The proposed degradation evaluation scheme of materials is shown in Figure 4.1. In vitro degradation studies often vary with the class of material, solvent, temperature, and duration. Solvents may include buffers at various pH values with or without enzymes and ions of elements that are expected to be present in and simulate the in vivo environment where the material or device will be used. Temperatures above the glass transition temperature may affect the crystallinity and rate of degradation of a polymer. Suggested accelerated temperatures for polymers are 50-80°C. The duration of an accelerated in vitro study is varying intervals up to 60 days whereas real-time tests at 37°C may extend up to 26 weeks. In either case, the solvent and device or material should be sterile to avoid confounding results from microbial contamination.

The solvent or extract from accelerated or real-time degradation exposure studies may additionally be subject to chemical and physical analyses. Analyses of polymers include identification of low molecular weight extractives, molecular weight changes of the polymer, viscosity measurements, thermal properties, changes in chemical structure, impurities, and changes on the material surface and within the bulk volume of the material. Degradation tests for ceramics, metals, and alloys in vitro generally emphasize quantification of the ions released into the solvent during the experiment and analyses for mass loss, compression strength, tensile strength, and surface properties by spectroscopic and microscopic methods.

Degradation studies in vivo focus on the implanted test sample and the adjacent tissues. Techniques that may be suitable depending upon the material include light microscopy, transmission electron microscopy, scanning electron microscopy; elemental analysis by electron probe analysis, neutron activation analysis, atomic absorption spectroscopy, inductively coupled plasma-mass spectroscopy, or microincineration of tissue(s) surrounding a metal implant; and organic chemical analyses by various chromatographic methods as gas-liquid chromatography, high performance liquid chromatography, and gel permeation chromatography. The selection of any of these methods will depend on the composition of the material, the detection and quantitation limits of the technique, and other factors. Analytical characterization of polymeric degradation is perhaps most advanced for the resorbable polyesters used for sutures. A mini-review of this topic is presented in the annexes of ISO 10993—Part 9.

Toxicokinetic Studies

ISO 10993 standard, Biological Evaluation of Medical devices—Part 16: Toxicokinetic Study Design for Degradation Products and Leachables was developed to evaluate the biological disposition of chemicals that may arise from extraction in vitro or biodegradation in vivo. Toxicokinetic studies determine the biological disposition of a foreign chemical whereas the term pharmacokinetics is applied when the substance being investigated is a pharmaceutical drug substance. Degradation products are the byproduct(s) of a material, which are generated by the breakdown or decomposition of the material. Leachables are the extractable component, such as additives, monomers, and low molecular weight constituents in polymeric materials. Toxicokinetic studies have historically been applied to resorbable materials to evaluate the disposition of the degradation products. More recently, these studies are being applied to chemicals that have been identified as extractives or degradation products from other medical devices. Examples include the sterilization agents as ethylene oxide and formaldehyde, xenograft cross-linking agents as glutaraldehyde, and mercury released from dental amalgams. More extensive use of these methods is expected in the future.

Toxicokinetic studies evaluate the kinetics of absorption, distribution, metabolism, and elimination of specific chemicals and are usually limited to studies of extractable chemicals or biodegradation products. Absorption is defined as when the chemical reaches the bloodstream. Thus, absorption studies are applicable to oral, inhalational, cutaneous, intracutaneous, mucosal, and implantation routes of exposure but not to vascular routes of exposure. Distribution studies determine the quantity of the chemical in the different tissues at various time intervals. Comparison of the concentration of the test substance in blood and tissues identifies accumulation in a specific tissue and the increased potential for toxic effects. Metabolism studies evaluate the enzymatic conversion of the agent to degradation products that may be further metabolized or excreted. Elimination studies evaluate the rate and routes of excretion. Toxicokinetic studies should define the mathematical model and method of calculating the half-lives for distribution and elimination and whether the elimination half-life is from blood, plasma, or total body elimination. Comparison of the plasma half-life with the tissue distribution also indicates potential for toxicity in those tissues where there is significant accumulation. If the studies involve tracking a radiolabelled molecule, then the results are expressed as mass equivalents of the parent compound.

Effectiveness Testing

Effectiveness testing from the perspective of regulated medical devices in the United States requires that the manufacturer demonstrate that the device meets the requirements of general controls, performance standards, or special controls. General controls are embodied in the Good Manufacturing Practices regulations [Part 21: U.S. Code of Federal Regulations (CFR), Section 211], quality assurance program of the individual manufacturer, and ISO 9000 and 14000 series of standards. Performance standards refer to guidance documents or standards developed for specific medical devices and are frequently available for class II and class III devices, i.e., those devices for which general controls are insufficient to provide reasonable assurance of safety and effectiveness (see Chapter 2). Examples of performance standards issued by FDA include guidance documents for longterm neurological implants, medical lasers, vascular grafts, testicular implants, breast implants, intra-articular knee ligament devices, metallic surface treated orthopedic implants fixed by tissue ingrowth, contact lenses, intraocular lenses, blood oxygenators, nondrug intrauterine devices, endosseous implants, bone anchor devices, replacement heart valves, and others. Additionally, FDA provides a catalog of medical device standards that have been published by various organizations and government agencies. This catalog, Medical Devices Standards Activities Report, is available from the FDA Center for Devices and Radiological Health, Office of Science and Technology, Standards Program Coordination Staff or through the Internet at http://www.fda.gov in the subfile Additional Sources of Information within the file Medical Device/Radiological Health. Special controls include, in addition to performance standards, controls such as postmarket surveillance, patient registries, guidelines, recommendations, and other appropriate actions deemed necessary by FDA.

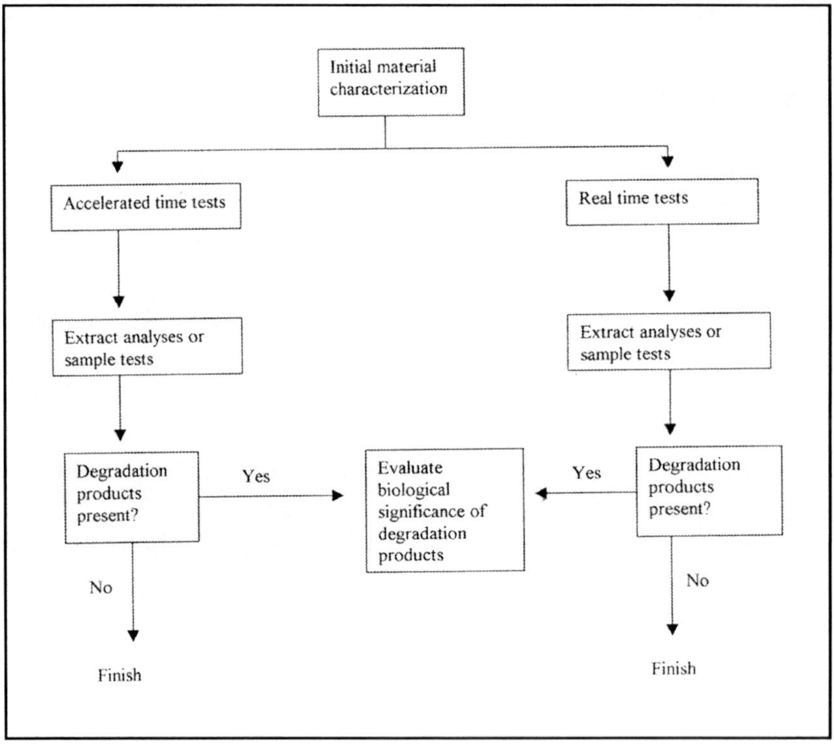

Fig. 4.1. Evaluation scheme for degradation studies.

The mechanisms for the establishment, amendment, or revocation of a performance standard or special control for a device are described in Part 21: U.S. CFR, Section 861.

The development of new medical devices is expected to follow the FDA's document, Design Control Guidance for Medical Device Manufacturers (Part 21: U.S. CFR, Section 820). Design control requirements are imposed on all class II, class III, and certain class I medical device manufacturers. The Guidance specifies preparation of a list of requirements to identify the performance characteristics of a medical device and confirmation by examination and objective evidence that specified requirements have been fulfilled. The elements of the list of performance requirements are unique for each device. Requirements might include the general controls of sterility, integrity, functionality of moveable parts, wear testing, component stress testing, failure mode analysis, and other verification activities, as appropriate. In the simplest sense, effectiveness testing of medical devices seeks to determine if the device does what it was designed to do. Some of the effectiveness testing focuses on physical and engineering tests to confirm that the device meets the performance requirements. Additional tests are conducted to identify failure modes using various scenarios that may occur under the usual and worst-case conditions of use.

Performance standards or special controls are often available for medical devices that have been marketed for an extended period. New or novel devices are unlikely to have product specific performance standards but would be expected to share some of the requirement criteria of other devices with similar attributes. However, it should be noted, device standards may not necessarily include all of the essential performance and effectiveness criteria for a given device.

This section presents case studies of performance and effectiveness criteria for three medical devices to illustrate the thoroughness and complexity of the process of developing criteria.

Externally Communicating Devices

Infusion sets are used for the administration of fluids intravenously to the clinical patient. The fluids infused through the set may be a caloric source such as glucose, electrolytes, nutrients, pharmacologically active drugs, or diagnostic agents. A flow pump, gravity feed, or pressure infusion may control the rate of infusion. The design for an infusion set includes the external and internal tubing diameter, length of tubing, type of connectors, materials of construction, drip chamber, additive port, flashball, spike, and other special features. Outputs from the design phase might include the architectural requirements, blueprints, subassemblies, dimensional tolerances for the components, functional specifications, and reliability requirements. Performance testing of prototypes during the development phase may include performance when used with an infusion pump, kinking of tubing, cracking of the spike and connectors, resealability of the additive port and flashball when punctured with a needle, leakage, flow rates, failure modes, integrity of the seals between the tubing and other components, compatibility with the sterilization agent or process, use of alcohol or other microbial decontamination agents during clinical use, compatibility with drugs that may be infused through the set, and other parameters. A protocol and report of testing for each of these criteria documents the performance effectiveness of the infusion set. At this phase of development, manufacturing documents are prepared and a manufacturing process validation protocol is written. Additionally, package design, qualification of vendors of components, and drafts of product labeling, user instructions, maintenance, and service manuals are produced. The validation protocol includes the design verification activities to be conducted on the first lot of manufactured product. Verification testing of the manufactured device demonstrates that the manufactured device meets the performance requirements of the design.

A FDA guidance document for hemodialyzer testing (1994) identifies key performance and efficacy testing for an ex vivo, externally communicating device that will be used clinically in intermittent, chronic applications. Since more than 70% of the hemodialysis facilities in the United States practice some form of dialyzer reprocessing and reuse, both new and approved hemodialyzers must be evaluated as to the limitations of reuse and the methods of performing safe and effective reprocessing. Effectiveness testing in vitro would include: volume of the blood compartment over the anticipated operating pressure ranges; pressure drop across the blood compartment as a function of minimum and maximum transmembrane pressures; changes in blood hematocrit during simulated hemodialysis; and pressure testing for blood leakage using a suitable dye. The pressure drop across the dialysate compartment as a function of dialysate flow, at minimum and maximum recommended transmembrane pressure, should be determined for high-permeability hemodialyzers. Effectiveness testing in vivo includes hemocompatibility, complement activation, urea clearance, blood pressure, hematocrit, and blood clotting, for example.

Implanted Devices

The guidance document for a vascular graft prosthesis includes performance and effectiveness criteria. Requirements listed in the guidance are porosity, water permeability, leakage, strength, suture retention strength, suture hole elongation, kink radius, crush resistance, durability, compliance, strength after repeated punctures, internal diameter, internal diameter under physiologic pressure, usable length, nominal wall thickness, assessment in animals, and clinical evaluation in humans for a particular clinical application. Physical testing must be performed on nine samples, with three samples from each of three lots. Durability testing determines the mechanical strength and compliance during which samples of the prosthesis are subjected to pulsatile pressure at a high frequency to simulate an extended period of implantation. Determination of strength after repeated puncture is evaluated to simulate dialysis access use of a vascular access device. Assessment in animals is based on the intended clinical application and the biological characteristics of the animal. The purpose is to evaluate the capacity of the prosthesis to maintain physiological function when used in the circulatory system, the response of the host animal, and the response of the prosthesis. Operative data requirements from the animal study are a description of the surgical procedure, type of proximal and distal anastomoses, immediate postoperative care, in situ length and diameter of the prosthesis, and adverse peri-operative events as transmural blood leakage. Functional assessment of graft performance might include patency assessment, angiography, ultrasonography, or other imaging techniques. Data at selected study intervals and termination include gross and microscopic pathology of the implantation site with representative photographs and micrographs, and physical analyses of the prosthesis for localized or diffuse dilatation, anastomotic disruption, thromboses and emboli, occlusion from other causes, infection, patency, or bleeding. The anastomosis between the vein and prosthesis is evaluated for abnormal healing, lumenal narrowing, stenosis, and other abnormalities. Radiographic studies are suggested to assess the extent of prosthesis calcification, if indicated. Electron microscopy may be warranted in specialized studies of the prosthesis fabric and its interactions with adjacent tissues.

Conclusion

This chapter reviewed the methods for nonclinical testing of medical devices for safety and effectiveness. Safety testing reviewed the general requirements for all medical devices and noted the common exceptions for highly specialized devices. Detailed methodologies of the in vitro and in vivo safety tests were discussed. The methods covered the generally accepted practices for cytotoxicity, immune sensitization, irritation, systemic toxicity, pyrogenicity, genotoxicity, implantation, hemocompatibility, chronic toxicity, carcinogenicity, reproductive effects, biodegradation, and toxicokinetics. The specific variables of these assays were designed to exaggerate the intended clinical use application. This exaggeration is achieved by either increasing the conditions of extraction, dose, rate of exposure, or using a test system that is more sensitive than the clinical population. Negative results in these assays or no observable adverse effects permit a qualitative hazard statement that the medical devices or materials are not predicted to cause adverse effects in humans because the assays are conducted at the biological or physiological limits of the test system. That is, any potential biological effects are below the detection limit of the assays.

Effectiveness testing consists of general controls, performance standards, or special controls which are embodied in a quality assurance program, guidance documents or standards for specific medical devices, design control requirements specified by the manufacturer, and postmarket surveillance, patient registries, guidelines, and others, where appropriate. Broadly defined, effectiveness testing includes physical and engineering tests for functionality and failure mode analyses as well as any testing in an animal model or during clinical trials.

The development of standards, guidances, design controls, and other documents serves a vital educational function for the medical device community. These documents represent the best-demonstrated practices and delineate the cumulative experiences of participating individuals. The tests described in these documents should be considered in the development of a medical device. Where appropriate, the rationale for omitting or deviating from the specified requirements should be documented. Additionally, it is to be anticipated that the art of safety and effectiveness testing will change with new knowledge and developments in improving biocompatibility.

References

1. Anonymous. F756 Standard Practice for assessment of hemolytic properties of materials. West Conshohocken, PA: ASTM. 1996.
2. Anonymous. Standard F0748, Practice for Selecting Generic Biological Test Methods for Materials and Devices. West Conshohocken, PA: ASTM. 1994.
3. Ashammaki NA. Neomembranes: A concept review with special reference to self-reinforced polyglycolide membranes. J Biomed Matr Res 1996; 33:297-303.
4. Benahmed M, Heymann D, Pilet P, Bienvenu J, Daculsi G. LPS increases biomaterial degradation by human monocytes in vitro. J Biomed Matr Res 1997; 34:115-119.
5. Brand KG, Buoen LC, Brand I. Carcinogenesis from polymer implants: new aspects from chromosome and transplantation studies during premalignancy. J Natl Cancer Inst 1967; 39:663-679.
6. Bush RB. A bibliography of monographic works on biomaterials and biocompatibility. J Appl Biomatr 1993; 4:195-209.
7. Chapman J, Lee W, Youkilis E, Martis L. Animal model for ethylene oxide (ETO) associated hypersensitivity reactions. Trans Am Soc Artif Intern Organs 1986; 32:482-485.
8. Didisheim P. 1997. Personal communication.
9. Food and Drug Administration (U.S.), Center for Devices and Radiological Health. Guidance for the preparation of research and marketing applications for vascular graft prostheses. Rockville, MD: Food and Drug Administration, Center for Devices and Radiological Health. 1993.
10. Food and Drug Administration (U.S.), Center for Devices and Radiological Health. RPTS Hemodialyzers: Guidance for testing. Guidance for hemodialyzer testing, with special instructions for reuse labeling. Rockville, MD: Food and Drug Administration, Center for Devices and Radiological Health. [Fifth Draft. March 14, 1994.]
11. Food and Drug Administration (U.S.), Center for Devices and Radiological Health. Design control guidance for medical device manufacturers. Rockville, MD: Food and Drug Administration, Center for Devices and Radiological Health. 1996.
12. Guidelines for blood/material interactions: Report of the National Heart, Lung, and Blood Institute. Working Group, U.S. Department of Health and Human Services, Public Health Service, National Institutes of Health NIH. Publication 85-2185. 1985.
13. Jarkelid L, Kjellstrand P, Marinson E, Wieslander, A. Toxicity of 20 chemicals from the MEIC programme determined by growth inhibition of L-929 fibroblast-like cells. ALTA 1997; 25:55-59.
14. Langone JJ. Immunotoxicity testing guidance. US Food and Drug Administration, Center for Devices and Radiological Health, Office of Science and Technology, Rockville, MD. Draft document April 6, 1998.
15. Maurin N, Daty N, Guerniew C, Dahmen K, Richter H. An in vivo study of the biodegradation of the hydrophilic Mitrathane®. J Biomed Matr Res 1997; 34:73-78.
16. Rao SB, Sharma CP. Use of chitosan as a biomaterial: Studies on its safety and hemostatic potential. J Biomed Matr Res 1997; 34:21-28.
17. Rockel A, Wahn V, Hertel J, Fiegel P. Ethylene oxide hypersensitivity reactions in dialysis patients. Lancet 1986; 1:382-383.
18. Stark NJ. Managing positive biocompatibility test results. Med Dev Diag Indust 1996; 18(10):148-162.
19. Tennant RW, Margolin BH, Shelby MD, Seiger E, Haseman JK, Spalding J, Caspary W, Resnick M, Stasiewicz S, Anderson B, Minor R. Prediction of chemical carcinogenicity in rodents from in vitro genetic toxicity assays. Sci 1987; 236:933-941.
20. Tripartite Biocompatibility Guidance for Medical Devices. U.S. Food and Drug Administration, Toxicology Subgroup of the Tripartite Subcommittee on Medical Devices. 1986.
21. US Food and Drug Administration, Center for Devices and Radiological Health, Rockville, MD. Immunotoxicity testing framework. Draft Oct. 28, 1996.
22. US Pharmacopeia. <85> Bacterial Endotoxins Test. US Pharmacopeia 2000; 24:1829-1831.
23. US Pharmacopeia. <151> Pyrogen Test. US Pharmacopeia 2000; 24:1850-1851.
24. US Pharmacopeia. <161> Transfusion and Infusion Assemblies. US Pharmacopeia 2000; 24:1851.

CHAPTER 5

Failure Analysis: Learning for the Future from the Past

Michael N. Helmus

One of the most important tasks a medical device manufacturer can make is to have a detailed methodology in place for explant analysis. The ability to examine the device for both adverse biological responses and for durability related to fatigue, corrosion, and degradation mechanisms is an important component of documenting the safety and efficacy of the device. It becomes critically important that all relevant information relating to the patient at implant, after implant, the time of the event and explant be documented. This includes patient health, medication pre-, peri-, postsurgery, activity, operating notes, x-rays, echos, MRI, and all relevant diagnostic testing. Table 5.1 outlines an approach to the decision making in developing an explant prototocol.

The concepts described here can be applied to both animal and human implants. With animal studies a complete and detailed protocol can be followed from implant through explant and analysis. Since animal studies can be well controlled, immunohistochemical analyses on fresh frozen tissue can be utilized in understanding biological responses including characterization of enzymes and cytokines present in the healing response. The use of immunohistochemistry is useful to characterize reactions to a particular disease state or inflammatory disease that may have resulted in excessive tissue formation, e.g., pannus on heart valves, stents, or grafts, or thrombosis. Unfortunately, many of the immunohistochemical agents will only be effective on human tissue, though there may be some cross-reactivity in certain animal models, particularly primates. Many times fresh frozen sections are impossible since the explants are not controlled in advance and samples are traditionally placed in formaldehyde solutions for fixation and to reduce risk of communicable disease. In many clinical explants the only controllable documentation and analysis occurs once the implant is brought into the lab performing the explant studies. Though it is often difficult to control how the device is removed, it is desirable to maintain the tissue/device interface. In a reoperation the chief criteria will be to preserve as much of the intact tissue and it may not be practical to maintain the interface. If the explant is done at autopsy in an institution that has a prior protocol, then removal of tissue adjacent to the device will be important in assessing local biological interactions. This is important in assessing hyperplastic responses that may occur in situations such as the anastomosis of devices, particularly in vascular tissue, pannus overgrowth of the sewing ring in heart valves and annuloplasty devices, and in balloon angioplasty, ablation angioplasty, and stenting, both in vascular and nonvascular applications (e.g., esophageal, tracheal, biliary). The device should be explanted into a fixative, e.g., a buffered formalin. A plan for physical examination and photography should be made including observations for thrombosis, fibrosis, infection, etc. After

Biomaterials in the Design and Reliability of Medical Devices, edited by Michael N. Helmus

Table 5.1 Approach to explant analysis[1]

Biologic Interactions			Material Properties
Implant History—device, patient/animal, medication (pre-, peri- , postoperative), patient history, removal history (revision, autopsy), gross photographs in situ and after removal (keeping device moist with saline and limiting time of exposure to air). Blood contacting devices can result in embolic episodes and organs such as the brain, lungs, and kidneys are particularly important to evaluate for infarcts. Device removal and handling as described below.			
Cell activity/metabolism **Cell types and receptors** **Enzyme, cytokines, growth factors** **Extracellular matrix composition** **Immunochemistry**	**Blood materials interaction** **Recellularization**	**Tissue interface and/or ingrowth** **Hyperplastic responses** **Tissue type (soft tissue, bone, neural, blood, etc)** **Extracellular matrix** **Cell type** **Cytomorphology**	**Material degradation** **Surface defects/degradation/cracking** **Wear**[2] **Crystal structure** **Crack initiation sites**
Cell isolation and purification **Thymidine uptake studies** **Fresh frozen sections with immunohistochemistry** **Special formalin fixatives**	**Extracorporeal devices** can be evaluated by changes in systemic parameters such as clotting time, hematological parameters, inflammation markers, and effects on lungs and kidneys. **Radiolabeled blood elements** can be useful to analyze blood element uptake and embolization in animal models. In rare circumstances these may be	**Paraffin sections** for traditional histology. **Hard sections** for bone and preserving tissue/device interface, particularly for bone and metallic implants. **Histologic stains** stains should be selected for cellular identification, e.g. H&E, extracellular matrix, e.g. Masson's Trichrome, or biologic responses such as calcification (e.g. Van Kossa 's stain). **Elemental analysis** (e.g., Energy dispersive analysis; electron diffraction; atomic adsorption) and TEM with osmium	After preparing samples for biologic evaluation, tissue removal with enzymes or hydroxides (see text) can be performed before or after fixation, except as noted. Tissue removal for bioprosthetic devices may be problematic. Table 1.6 outlines material evaluations for biostability including **molecular weight** measurements. If samples are large enough, **mechanical properties** can be evaluated by tensile testing or small samples by dynamic mechanical analysis. Changes in properties may also be seen by **shrink temperature** of collagen based materials if fresh explant or changes in **thermal properties** e.g., glass transition or melt temperature in polymers. Reflected light **microscopy** with or without

Table 5.1. Approach to explant analysis[1] (continued)

Biologic Interactions			Material Properties
	used clinically. **Scanning electron microscopy** for surface cellular interactions e.g., endothelialization, epithelialization, etc. requires the use of osmotically balanced glutaraldehyde buffers.	tetroxide staining for **cytomorphology**.	special optics (e.g., polarizing lenses, differential interference contrast) and SEM are particularly useful. **Profilometry** of wear depths might be considered. **Elemental analysis** can be performed by energy dispersive analysis or whole microprobe on whole samples. Atomic adsorption can be used on dissolved samples. **Metallography/structure** related to processing, crystal size, voids, defects, inclusions that can relate to initiation of fatigue cracking.

[1] All explants require handling as a biohazard material. This is particularly of concern with human and primate tissue that can harbor human pathogens. Fresh tissue requires extra care as no fixatives are used. Fixatives reduce but may not eliminate the chance of transmission, therefore all tissue should be handled as as a biohazard.
[2] These evaluations are appropriate for explants as well as devices subjected to accelerated wear/durability testing.

thorough documentation, the device and tissue samples for histological, scanning electron microscopy (SEM), and potentially transmission electron microscopy* would be selected. General histologic stains, like H&E are useful for general cellular interaction. Specific stains for extracellular matrix, e.g., Trichrome for collagen and Von Giesson's stain for elastin are useful. References are available that review suitable stains for particular identificiation of extracellular matrix and cells.[1,12,14] Histologic analysis of fibroproliferative disease treatment, e.g., restenosis after angioplasty or stenting and anastomotic intimal hyperplasia in vascular grafting, is an important method of analysis in order to determine the effectiveness of treatments with respect to cellular proliferation and extracellular matrix formation. Treatments based on energy methods and drug delivery methods target inhibition of smooth muscle cells in this process.

SEM analysis of biologic tissue may require preservation in an osmotically balanced glutaraldehyde or paraformaldehyde fixative.[12] This is generally not performed unless the particular institution is prepared for these types of analyses in advance. SEM is extremely useful for documenting cellular responses and thrombus formation on surfaces as well as documenting the nature of the surface texture or for surface defects. Certain materials and devices may require the use of epoxy embedding and thin sectioning in order to preserve the tissue/device interface for histological analysis. This method may be employed in endovascular stents and stent graft applications where the material is a metal tissue interface[1a] and cannot be processed by traditional embedding in paraffin. Fabric tissue interfaces can be processed by traditional methods but requires some art in order to preserve the interfaces.

Observation of the integrity of the underlying device substrate may require the tissue to be removed, as discussed below, so surfaces can be examined for defects as well as damage that may have been caused by rough handling or surgical instrumentation at the time of use/implantation. The device can be cleaned of biologic deposits using enzymes or hydroxides.[3,5,8,9] After cleaning a thorough observation and microscopy for mechanical integrity can be made. Critical components can be examined, e.g., mechanical fittings, pivot points, etc. If a crack or fractured surface is found, SEM or replicas of the surface should be made. Morphology with relation to crack initiation or type of crack propagation may be possible. Wear mechanisms, important in orthopedic joint implants and mechanical heart valves, can be documented.

Critical material components can be sampled for physiochemical testing to demonstrate if changes in material properties have occurred. If properties are not durable in the way anticipated in the design, failure could result. This can be true with respect to strength, stiffness, lubricity, dimensional stability, etc.

In the design process a comprehensive study of design, durability, and animal explant analysis can be designed from the start. The proposed design needs to be evaluated for potential failure modes. For example, at sites where components are joined, finite element modeling might be appropriate to study stresses expected at that site. For devices that are constantly flexed, modeling based on known fatigue properties are appropriate. After the modeling the actually fabricated component should be tested for their ability to meet these design requirements prior to the full development process. Complex devices such as hip prostheses fixed with bone cement will need to evaluate failure modes in the cemented configuration, while coated prostheses, e.g., with hydroxyapatite, will need to evaluate failure due to coating degradation or delamination. Significant efforts have been extended in studying the fatigue properties of bone cements.

Durability is a measure of the lifetime of the device and is a measure not only of the fatigue characteristics under simulated physiologic conditions (life-testing) but of the biostability of the device under these conditions. Tests performed in labs measure fatigue in buffered

* Identification of cell types and the nature of the cell cytohistochemistry.

solutions. This can meaure, to some degree, corrosive and hydrolytic contributions to durability. However, degradation from lytic-enzymes, absorption, plasticizaton, and swelling by lipids and proteins, and the variation of pH and concentration of enzymes as a function of biologic interactions (e.g., acute infection, thrombosis, and chronic infection) cannot be measured in these systems. Alternative test methodologies to address biostability are necessary and include implants of materials under stress[13] to accelerate degradative mechanisms or an in vitro approach as outlined in Table 1.6.

Life testing is a critical aspect of the testing of devices that carry stress or are repetitively stressed during use. These can include orthopedic joint replacements, vascular grafts, heart valves, artificial hearts, intraaortic balloon pumps and pacemaker leads. This type of predictive testing is important since most animal tests are short term, e.g., 6 months to 1 year, and may not demonstrate failures that will occur at 5-10 years.

Durability as a function of stress-level is highly dependent on the application, namely how the stress is applied and the level of stress. In cardiovascular applications, heart valves, intraaortic balloon pumps and the artificial heart represent demanding cases. Failures have been observed in heart valve struts that experience stresses beyond that predicted by theoretical stress analysis. Finite element modeling can be extremely useful for assessing new designs and materials. This is potent when combined with testing to measure in situ stresses and with accelerated durability testing, e.g., testing of heart valves in aqueous solutions at a high rate of pulsing in order to test for years of use in short periods of time. This type of testing must not change the failure mode due to heat build up or variant closure of the leaflets. For example, accelerated fatigue testing that has loading in the accelerated condition different than in physiologic loading conditions can lead to erroneous conclusions, either predicting shorter or longer lives. Reul[7] suggests measuring loading conditions by use of instrumented device (e.g., strain gauges) or by measurement of unique characterisitics of the device (e.g., closing velocity of the leaflets in mechanical heart vlaves). Evaluation of orthopedic joints need to account for dynamic impacts, e.g., walking, running, jumping, and stair climbing, in the types of repetitive stressing that might occur over the lifetime of the device.

Prediction of failure in metallic devices and pyrolytic carbon components used in heart valves can be performed by either traditional fatigue analysis or by the damage tolerant approach. Both methods require that the stress state within the device is known so that the peak stress and stress state are known. Finite element modeling has been useful in determination of these states. Verification by strain gauging the device and experimental verification in vitro and in vivo is desirable. The classic approach to fatigue is based on stress-life, i.e., number of cycles to fatigue (S/N). This approach assumes that the defects that lead to crack propagation need to be initiated and grow to the size at which fracture will occur.[10] In the damage tolerance approach, it is assumed that the cracks already exist in the material and that the time to fatigue failue is the time it takes to propagate these inherent cracks to the critical sizes required for failure.[15] The approach can also be utilized to back calculate from the desired life time to the initial crack size that would produce this lifetime. This approach is considered relatively conservative since it ignores crack inititation. The ability to calculate crack sizes under which failure would not occur in a desired device lifetime allows the use of diagnostic techniques to measure acceptable crack size.

SN methods require that test components have the same properties as the components so that fatigue properties are representative of the device. The damage tolerant approach requries that inspection techniques can identify cracks sizes larger than the allowable initial crack size. Methods to do this involve dye penetrants, x-ray, eddy currents, and proof tesing. Proof testing has been used extensively with pyrolytic carbon components of heart valves. This tests each component by applying a stress that will cause brittle failure if a crack larger than acceptable exists in the component. Accurate descriptions of fatigue generally require the testing to be performed in buffered solutions since water and ions, in particular chloride, can accelerate crack growth by mechanisms such as stress-corrosion cracking.

The fatigue analyses work well for most metallic alloys, ceramics, and engineering plastics. However, the predictive nature of these studies isnot as suited to many polymeric materials and require testing in simulated physiologic environments. Accelerated conditions of fatigue can be utilized as long as failure mechanisms are not changed. For example, excessive heating leading to a temperature rise above a thermal transition like the glass transition temperature would potentially invalidate the test. Durability testing for many devices are required in addition to the fatigue analyses to demonstrate the essential safety of the device.

Many of the test methodologies for specific devices are outlined in the FDA Guidelines for specific devices. For example the heart valve guideline specifies the fracture mechanics approach for predicting lifetime of pyrolytic carbon heart valves.

References

1. Anderson JA. In: Cardiovascular Biomaterials and Biocompatibility. Harker LA, Ratner BD, and Didisheim P, eds. Supplement, Cardiovascular Pathology 1993; 2:199-216.
1a. Ding N, Helmus MN. Drug release coated stent, International Patent Application. PCT/IB96 00272, April 1, 1996.
2. Coury AJ, Slaikeu PC, Cahalan PT et al. Factors and interactions affecting the performance of polyurethane elastomers in medical devices. J Biomaterials Applications 1988; 3:130-179.
3. Couture J, Guidoin R, King M et al. Textile teflon arterial porstheses: How successful are they? Canadian J Surgery 1984; 27:575-582.
4. Gibbons DF. Material analysis of retrieved implants. In: Short Course, Evaluation and Testing of Cardiovascular Devices, June 12-13, 1995, Helmus MN, Chair; Coury AJ, CoChair; Society for Biomaterials. Course Notebook 1995, Cerritos, CA.
5. Guidoin R, Marceau D, Rao TJ et al. In vitro and in vivo characterization of an impervious polyester arterial prosthesis: The gelseal triaxial graft. Biomaterials 1987; 8:433-441.
6. Helmus M, Botan EA, Malone J et al. Sterility and pyrogenicity issues of synthetic vascular grafts, In: Kambic H, Kantrowitz A, Sung P, eds. Vascular Graft Update, ASTM Spec. Tech Publ. STP 898, Phila.:American Society for Testing and Materials, 1986:236-249.
7. Reul H, Eihler M, Potthast K, Schmitz C, Rau G. In Vitro Testing of Heart Valve Wear Outside of the Manufacturers Laboratory Requirements and Controversies. J Heart Valve Dis 5(I):97-104.
8. Maarek JM, Guidoin RM, Aubin RE. Molecular weight characterization of virgin and explanted polyester arterial prostheses, J Biomed Mater Res 1984; 18:881-894.
9. Needham DK, Buchanan DR, Horton HR et al. Enzymatic Removal of Formalin-Fixed Tissue from Polyester Arteries and Its Effect on Physical Properties, 39th Annual Tech Conf of Soc Plas Eng May 1981.
10. Ritchie RO. Fatigue and Fracture of Pyrolytic Carbon: A Damage-Tolerant Approach to Structural Integrity and Life Prediction in "Ceramic" Heart Valve Prostheses. J Heart Valve Dis 5, (Supplement I):9-31.
11. Stokes KB. Polyether polyurethanes, biostable or not? J Biomaterials Applications 1988; 3:228-259.
12. Schoen FJ. Interventional and Surgical Cardiovascular Pathology. Philadelphia: W.B.Saunders 1989; 268:124-171.
13. Szycher M. Biocompatible Polymers, Metals and Composites. Lancaster, Pa: Technomic Publishing 1983; 239-262, 395-406, 427-461, 477-523.
14. von Recum AF. Handbook of Biomaterials Evaluation, Scientific, Technical, and Clinical Testing of Implant Materials. New York: Macmillan Publishing Co. 1986:159-208.
15. Kafesjian R, Schmidt P. Life Analysis and Testing, Short Course, Evaluation and Testing of Cardiovascular Devices, June 12-13, 1995, M.N. Helmus Chair, A.J. Coury, Co-Chair, Society for Biomaterials, Course Notebook. 1995: Cerritos, CA.

CHAPTER 6

Product Development in a Small Company Environment

Roger W. Snyder

A small company, particularly a start-up operation, is an exciting, and often stressful, environment. If the company has a limited number of products, all under development, there is always pressure to get those products to market as soon as possible to generate sales and income. If the new device is also a new concept, the excitement of developing the product adds to the feeling of urgency.

In this environment of excitement and pressure, it is easy to concentrate on the day-to-day problems and difficult to look ahead. However, decisions made in the early phases of product development can have major impact on the success of product commercialization. Neglecting to initiate certain tasks early in the development process can significantly increase the time (and the cost) of getting your device to market. We discuss a number of case histories in this article that illustrate this point. These examples are real, but are not intended to be all-inclusive. They are used to illustrate pitfalls that small companies have encountered.

Much of the data required for patent filings and FDA applications are completed during the early phases of product development. Some of this same data is also useful for specification development, process validation, and possibly in future lawsuits. One of the most important and most overlooked aspects of product development in a small company environment is good record keeping. In the rush to fabricate samples of a new product and to develop the necessary processes, it is tempting to skip the recording of experiments and proposed design specifications. This missing information may be important at a later date. The risk of losing valuable information is high. The time required to get a product to market can actually be lengthened. since experiments will have to be repeated if pertinent information is missing.

There are two levels of testing generally undertaken during the development of a new product. First is the testing of samples to zero in on the desired prototype. The second level of effort involves testing of a prototype that is (or is close to) the final design. It is important to distinguish between the two levels. In the case of testing a prototype, characterization of the sample, defined test protocols, and thorough record keeping is extremely important. The benefits of careful testing of prototypes are often not apparent until much later in the product life cycle, when it is too late to retrieve meaningful results.

It is often difficult for small companies to obtain the necessary materials and components. A developer often uses samples in the early stages of product development, since the prototypes may change rapidly and may not represent the final product. However, you must be careful using samples. These samples may not represent the vendor's actual production, or may have deteriorated or have been damaged if they were used as demonstration samples. If it is necessary

Biomaterials in the Design and Reliability of Medical Devices, edited by Michael N. Helmus

to purchase components in larger than required quantities, use caution in labeling and storing leftover material. Avoid materials and components, whenever possible, that are difficult to get or traditionally have long lead times.

Recent advances in the art of fabricating prototypes, fueled by the desire of large companies to shorten design cycles, can be very beneficial to small companies. A company can significantly decrease the time to produce prototypes by using computer aided design programs (CAD), computer aided machining (CAM), rapid prototyping, and electronic data transfer. The use of express delivery services and facsimile machines decreases the time required to exchange information with consultants and vendors.

Good vendor relationships can be the life blood of a small company. The ability to get materials and supplies in small quantities, and to get rapid service, can be enhanced when a vendor feels that he or she is a part of the development effort. Often, discussing the company's products and goals (without, of course, divulging confidential information) can result in opening up vital lines of communication between your company and an important vendor. Vendors can also serve as sources of information concerning new products and future developments in areas of interest to the company.

Sterilization and shelf life testing are among the long lead time items that must be completed for successful product development. Choose an appropriate sterilization method early in the development phase in order to select appropriate materials for the design and the packaging and to prepare samples for other tests.

Once you have developed and tested prototypes, you need to plan and develop the facilities for the fabrication of the clinical or commercial samples. These facilities can range from designated storage and fabrication areas to clean rooms; depending upon the volume and type of product being manufactured. The facility design can be adversely impacted by decisions made during the early phases of product development.

Records and Record Keeping

It is difficult to take time to write down and organize results in the press of daily fire fighting. However, you may lose important test parameters and observations if you do not record them soon after the event. It will be easier to use the data in any future legal or regulatory activity if that information is complete and organized. A minimum requirement for this record keeping is a carefully maintained laboratory notebook.

The FDA has added a requirement for a design history to the Good Manufacturing Practices (GMP) regulation. This requirement was effective June 1997 and was being fully enforced as of June 1998. In addition, a design history is currently a requirement for product registration in the European Common Market. Thus laboratory test records become even more important. Both FDA audits (under the new GMP regulations) and audits for a European CE Mark will focus on the design history procedure itself and not on the data. However, well kept and organized data is one sign of a thorough design history process. Furthermore, an FDA audit in support of a PreMarket Approval (PMA) Application will focus on data review. Data that is accurate and organized will simplify the process of supporting a PMA.

Organized records could also be important for legal reasons. These documents may contain important examples for possible patent applications and may demonstrate the history of the development of a patentable idea. If faced with a product liability suit, these records may be useful to demonstrate due diligence in product design and testing. These records may also prove useful in protecting trade secrets should employees leave the company. They may provide information in the defense of lawsuits for trade secret infringement by previous employers.

Finally, a well-organized design history record provides a historical perspective for product and process changes. This perspective could include a demonstration of which variables are important and which play a minor role in maintaining product specifications. You can use the original test protocols to test changes in product or process parameters. The resulting data, when compared to the original tests, could support claims of an insignificant modification.

A design history record should contain the following five parts:

Design and development planning;
: a procedure describing authority and responsibility for product design (a simple plan would suffice for a small organization).

Design requirements;
: the proposed operating parameters and specifications (including those necessary to achieve a safe and efficacious performance of the device).

Design verification;
: test methods and results to verify that the design meets the previously approved design requirements.

Design output;
: formal release of a design to production (an approved Device Master Record).

Design changes;
: written documentation of any changes in the approved design.

Case History #1

An engineer who was responsible for the development of a new product for a small start-up operation was sued by his former employer. The law suit claimed that he used confidential information in developing the process for the new device. The engineer produced a number of patents, technical manuals and other documents describing the process. He also produced a description of his process compared to the process of his former employer. Finally, he produced his laboratory notebook.

The notebook contained notes from meetings, thoughts on product requirements, concepts and some important references. These notes might have been adequate to meet the first two requirements of a design history (for a small company with one engineer, the procedure for product design is simple). Unfortunately, the notebook did not document all of the testing that led up to the final prototype. This made it more difficult to demonstrate how the process could have been developed from public information.

The outcome of the lawsuit was a temporary injunction against the start-up company. We can not know what led to the judge's decision or whether or not additional data would have changed the outcome. However, it is possible that this data would have been useful for the defense. In addition, the data would have been useful in setting up a process validation protocol.

Case History #2

A start-up operation was formed to develop and market a product requiring a PreMarket Approval to commercialize. This product had both old and new indications. Several engineers and technicians did the initial development work. Because of the time required to complete the clinical testing, the PMA Application was submitted to the FDA several years after the completion of the original bench testing. The company also relocated twice within this period.

Once the FDA accepted the PMA, the Agency visited the company for a GMP audit as part of the PMA approval process. Toward the end of the two week audit, the field agent requested to see the original data sheets for the information in the PMA application. It took some time to locate the original notes. Most of the notes were on individual sheets of paper with little explanation or other details. When the condition of the data was noted, the auditor decided to review the information closely. The auditor compared each set of data in the PMA application to the notes and checked all of the calculations. A number of errors were found, particularly in the calculations. The company was forced to file an amendment to its PMA application and to its IDE before continuing the clinical study. Fortunately, the corrected data altered only one of the conclusions. The company was able to repeat the measurements for that conclusion.

The exercise delayed the company a month. However, if it had been necessary to repeat all of the testing, significant time would have been lost. As discussed, it is important to keep complete, organized, and accurate records of experiments. It is also important to check the data generated and the calculations.

Testing

Testing is required in a number of areas during the development phase of a medical device. Data to demonstrate the safety and the efficacy of the device must be gathered. This validation of the design may include bench testing, animal testing and clinical studies. Verification that the design meets the original design requirements (see Records and Record keeping) may require different testing than the device validation studies. Any software the device uses will also have to be validated. Tests will be required to demonstrate that the software (and the combination of the software and hardware) will yield the desired results under all inputs.

The processes needed to produce the device must also be validated, in particular, those processes whose output cannot be verified by testing (see, for example, Sterilization and Shelf Life). This testing requires manufacturing multiple lots of products, which increases the expense of testing. Thus this phase is normally completed after the design is finalized. The products sampled for process validation can often be used for clinical studies or be sold.

It is important to distinguish between the two types of samples normally tested during the product development phase: early prototypes and final design prototypes. During the early stages of development, rapid turnover is important. Testing should be adequate to provide direction for the development process. Testing of final design prototypes should demonstrate that the design meets the design specifications.

As discussed previously, careful recording of the data, even in the early stages of development, is important. Often this data is key in making future changes in the design or process. Also, this information often establishes a data trail in case of future regulatory or legal actions.

What distinguishes testing done in the early stages of development from what is done on later stages is the amount of sample characterizations done and numbers of samples tested. Since it is necessary to make rapid progress in the early stages of development, large numbers of samples are usually not available for testing. However, you should take every care that the results obtained are representative. Written test protocols and the use of certified or calibrated instruments are highly recommended.

As the samples approach the desired final design characteristics, the nature of testing should change. More and more information about the test samples is required. Process records (lot histories) should be maintained, particularly if the resulting data will be submitted to a regulatory agency. Product specifications and process parameters should have tolerances where possible. Use at least 3 representative samples in any significant test. A sample size that would yield statistically significant results would be preferable. A carefully written test plan may permit several tests to be carried out on the same set of samples, particularly if you carry out destructive tests last.

At this stage, all tests should be done to written protocols. Consideration should be given to having important tests (for example, tests to confirm compliance with standards such as UL requirements) done by an accredited laboratory. You will also have to contract out tests requiring specialized equipment or facilities (for example, biocompatibility studies). Select and treat these laboratories just as you would any other vendor (see discussion below).

Samples sent to laboratories should be characterized. Sample characterization should include a description of the sample (including materials used) and the sample's processing history. Data on samples used for biocompatibility studies should also include bulk and surface chemistry, and possible leachates.

Check all test results, including those obtained in-house. Audit reports for accurate conclusions, signatures and the presence of extraneous comments that could mislead the reader. Check calculations for correctness (in terms of arithmetic, methods used and number of significant digits reported). Compare results to expected outcomes and similar data. Investigate any unexpected results. Justify, appropriately, the omission of any data from the reported results.

The FDA requires that data demonstrating product safety be done under Good Laboratory Practices (GLP's). These regulations are similar to GMP's, requiring an approved protocol, written procedures, control of samples, and an independent quality control unit. Adherence to the protocol and procedures is to be verified and all data is to be reviewed by this quality control unit. Well-run laboratories will have protocols, procedures, and sample control. There is usually an extra charge to perform studies under GLP regulations; primarily due to the extra labor involved with the quality control unit. Whether or not a study is important enough to perform under GLP regulations is a management decision that should be discussed with the laboratory performing the work.

Case History #3

A start-up operation was developing a cleaning process for an implant. The company chose a local laboratory to do the testing because of the potential number of samples and the desire for rapid turn-around of results. This laboratory specialized in environmental testing, standard EPA tests, analysis of residues, and fire investigation. The need for a rapid test capable of detecting low levels of wetting agents and contaminants was discussed with the lab director. He recommended a Total Organic Carbon analysis that would be a measure of the contamination on the product. Samples were extracted in deionized water using a Soxhlet extractor by the company. The laboratory then determined the TOC level in each sample.

The company initially tried a large number of process variations. Three samples per variation were prepared and tested. Three extraction stations were set up so that creating multiple samples did not cost any additional time. Care had to be taken not to contaminate the extraction, either in preparation of the sample or in loading the extract into the analyzer. The experiment was repeated if the result from one of the samples did not agree with the other two. This happened several times. Using three samples avoided eliminating a promising process improvement.

Once the desired final result was obtained, the proposed process was run three consecutive times. Three samples were prepared and tested for each run. This more extensive test documented the variation from run to run, as well as from sample to sample. It also established a baseline for future process validation studies in which process tolerances were tested.

Samples were also processed for biocompatibility studies. A TOC analysis was completed on these samples as well. In addition, the process developer completed other extraction tests, sent samples out for infrared spectrophotometry scans and measured all important dimensions. Using this graduated approach, the company was able to develop a process in a minimum amount of time. Sample size was adequate to detect experimental errors. The more detailed safety studies carried out on the final process were adequate to demonstrate safety to the appropriate regulatory agencies.

Materials and Components

It is often difficult for small companies to obtain the materials and components necessary to fabricate prototypes. The short lead times and small quantities necessary for product development make it difficult to acquire many items. This is especially true for materials that are normally sold in bulk (such as plastic resins and dyes), as well as components that have long lead times (such as specialized electronic parts).

The most common way to get around this problem is to use samples. However, it is important to be sure that these samples are truly representative of the vendor's product. A vendor may ship a potential customer a representative product for evaluation. A product developer can also obtain samples from a salesperson. These samples could be loaners or materials used to demonstrate product features. Sometimes these samples are products that did not meet original specifications, and were set aside for the sales force. The samples may have been damaged by repeated demonstrations (or while stored in the salesperson's car trunk). Finally, a sample may have used up its useful shelf life or, even worse, could be obsolete.

An alternative to using samples is to locate another vendor who uses the same materials or components. For example, if you have tubing extruded by a vendor specializing in extrusion, or a part molded by a vendor specializing in ejection molding, they may be able to order small quantities of resins, or use a particular resin for several jobs. Similarly, a vendor specializing in assembling electronics may be able to get better service from an electronics parts supply house than your smaller order would get you.

Acquisition of large samples, particularly of bulk items, such as resins, leads to another potential problem. Many of these materials have specified shelf lives and/or recommended storage conditions. Between the time early prototypes are completed and the time arrives to fabricate final prototypes for testing, the materials or components could have deteriorated or corroded, particularly if improperly stored.

Establish a receiving procedure in the beginning. At the very least this should include a method to log in all incoming materials and components. This log should include vendors' names, description of the item, any vendor's part numbers, and lot numbers or serial numbers. In addition to the incoming material log, a vendor log should also be established. This log should note each vendor's performance, including timely delivery, quality of the material as received, and any problems experienced with the vendor. The information will help in qualifying vendors for future production items, which is a requirement under GMP and ISO 9000 regulations.

Inspect all key items as they arrive. If uninspected material is placed in storage and a flaw or defect is discovered when the item is used, it will be too late to get the vendor to take corrective action. Should a component with an unknown defect be used in a prototype, it may be difficult to determine why the prototype does not work. On the other hand, should the prototype be made to work in spite of the defective component, it may not be possible to duplicate the prototype or repeat the test data at a later date.

Case History #4

A small company wanted to design a second family of catheters. The CEO selected polymers and additives that he had gotten as samples several years previously. The catheter tubing was extruded and appeared to meet the design requirements. The same process developed for the company's original product was used to fabricate several prototypes. These catheters were shown to several physicians, who indicated that the product met their needs and they would participate in a clinical study.

Additional lots were fabricated from the same tubing. Samples were tested according to the applicable FDA Guideline. The catheters had inadequate tensile and burst strength. A microscopic examination of the failures indicated the presence of large particles in the tubing. Some of these particles were as large as one half of the tubing wall thickness. Investigation showed that these particles came from one of the additives. Thus the company would have to extrude new tubing. When the engineers went to order a replacement for that additive, the material was no longer available.

A substitute material was located and new tubing extruded. Once again samples were fabricated and tested. These samples now met all of the physical design requirements. It was not known if the sample additive came with the large particles or if the material clumped together in storage. There was no receiving information or data available for the sample. The material had been stored on a shelf in a back room with no climate control. What was obvious, however, was that a month had been lost in the product development process.

Prototyping

Unlike the problems faced by small companies in acquiring materials and components, acquiring machined and molded parts has gotten considerably easier in recent years. Because of the desire of many large corporations to shorten the product development process, there are now a large number of small companies that specialize in rapid turn around of molded plastic parts. These entrepreneurs use a variety of techniques including stereolithography, numerically controlled machining of aluminum master molds, plaster casting, reaction injection molding, etc. It is possible to produce plastic parts with a finished look in weeks instead of months. The same numerically controlled machining techniques can produce accurately machined metal parts in a similarly short period of time.

Today, the greatest delay in getting parts fabricated usually results from the difficulty of getting your job scheduled by the vendor. Many of the best shops have a constant backlog of work. As discussed in more detail in the next section, it is very helpful to establish good relations with a local machine shop. This can facilitate getting rush jobs completed expeditiously or can result in receiving helpful suggestions on a tricky design issue.

Advancements in electronic communications have also improved prototype turn around. Transmission of data (such as drawings) electronically to a suitably equipped machine shop can significantly cut the time required to machine a part or mold. Transmission can be done via a modem or on a floppy disk or tape. Even the use of a FAX can save time, particularly in the signing of contracts or confidentiality agreements. It is also possible to transmit text via the internet. You can send software to a vendor for validation using this technology.

Of course, to make full use of these advancements, a company must invest in computers, modems, faxes, etc. Fortunately, the price of electronic devices is falling, allowing even the smallest company to participate in the information age. Small companies must also locate prototyping shops and machine shops that can work with the types of data the company's equipment can generate and who are willing to work with small companies.

As a particular design approaches maturity, avoid using items around the lab (such as old adhesives, unmarked screws, pieces of scrap metal or plastic, etc.) to solve problems or produce new prototypes. The use of materials from unknown sources will complicate repeating results, writing specifications, and transferring the design to production. It is also important to fabricate and test prototypes in an environment that will not affect the test results. For example, samples intended for biocompatibility should not be fabricated in a dirty area where the samples would be contaminated. On the other hand, these samples should not be cleaned beyond what would be expected in production. Either extreme may yield erroneous results.

Finally, problems with a design invariably occur. It is important to understand the cause of a particular problem, before developing and applying a solution. Otherwise, the solution can create new unwanted problems. A design with multiple patches often results from solving a series of problems. Such a design is not robust and is often difficult to manufacture.

Case History #5

Fifteen years ago a small company needed to get plastic cases fabricated for a medical device going into a clinical study. The original prototypes were machined out of solid blocks of hard plastic. The resulting cases were too heavy and too costly. Investigation showed that it would take 12 to 16 weeks to get a mold machined for an ejection molded case. It would then take another 4 to 6 weeks to get the parts molded. Even an aluminum mold designed for low production quantities would be costly (in time and money). The company went to a vendor who specialized in rapid turn around prototypes. The vendor machined a male mold out of aluminum and fabricated silicone female molds. Cases could be fabricated at a rate of 2 or 3 a day using liquid casting techniques. This was adequate for the quantities required. In 4 weeks, parts were available suitable for use in a clinical study.

Recently, another start-up company required a similar case in small quantities for testing and a clinical study. The designers used a popular CAD drafting program to provide electronic drawings to a local vendor. Using stereolithography, the vendor formed the male mold directly from the electronic drawings. The rest of the process was similar to the one described above. Parts were available in 1 week.

The drawback of these procedures is the requirement to use liquid castable materials. The strength of these materials and their ability to withstand high temperatures are somewhat limited. When you design with these materials, these limitations must be taken into account. However, the ability to get parts fabricated in a short time period can be a major benefit to a design project, particularly if changes in these parts are required as the design matures.

Vendor Relationships

Careful selection of vendors can make a difference between the success and failure of a small company. Close relationships with key vendors (or their representatives) can yield improved service, furnish early warnings of new or soon to be discontinued products, and provide information on industrial and regulatory trends.

Where possible, use vendors or consultants with proven records. Vendors who are also medical device companies must be registered with the FDA and must have a Quality Assurance program. Recently, ISO 9000 certification has become popular. An ISO 9000 certified company will also have an active Quality Assurance program. A registered auditor will audit these companies every year or so. Some large corporations (such as the automotive companies) also audit their vendors, as do many medical device companies. You can check credit references and references from satisfied customers. Finally, there are a number of independent laboratory accreditation programs that require meeting certain standards. A vendor should be willing to document compliance with any of these programs.

Where possible, key vendors should be visited. Viewing the vendor's facility and reviewing their quality control program can also provide assurances as to the vendor's capability and desire to meet specifications and commitments. This visit may also help to establish a good relationship with a particular vendor.

As discussed under Materials and Components, a history of vendor performance (based on receiving records) will provide valuable information when qualifying a source. An approved vendor list can be established based on audits of key suppliers, or the vendor history accumulated during product development. It can also be based on contracts with vendors indicating a willingness to meet specifications, evidence of unsuccessful attempts to contact a supplier, or evidence that this vendor is a sole source supplier.

You can use certificates of compliance to receive materials and components, provided that you or your designate have audited the supplier's quality control program. This is another reason for visiting key suppliers. Otherwise, you (or an independent laboratory) must test incoming items in house, or use actual data supplied by the vendor.

Developing a good relationship with key vendors may be very beneficial to the product development effort. Vendors can be a valuable source of information about new developments, particularly in their area of expertise. They may be more willing to expedite an order or provide alternative methods to achieve a particular result.

A small company has a more difficult time working with vendors than do larger companies. A small company represents only a small volume of business to the vendor. Also, a vendor can anticipate that a long time will typically pass before a product will be commercialized. Therefore, a start up operation must make a special effort to develop a selection of reliable vendors. Take time to discuss the goals of the development effort (including soliciting and listening to the vendor's ideas). Also, keep a vendor informed as to progress (particularly in areas involving their products or services). Finally, negotiate fair contracts (benefiting both parties).

Case History #6

A start-up company (first discussed in Case History #5) made an effort to establish good relationships with the prototyping vendor. The vendor's sales engineer visited the company and was shown around the laboratory. His suggestions on how to maximize the benefits of the vendor's technology were utilized. The company audited the vendor (even though it required a trip half way across the country). A presentation of the product and its purposes was made to some of the vendor's personnel. The required quality for the product was discussed with the vendor's Quality Control Department. The company permitted the vendor to use the company's name and product in an article describing the vendor's technology.

The company had to redesign a second component of the device. The new design required radiation sterilization (because of the presence of a blind chamber). When the vendor was approached about the possibility of liquid casting this device, neither the company nor the vendor knew of a radiation resistant castable plastic. However, the vendor called a number of his contacts and his vendors and was able to locate a material that met all of the design's requirements. The vendor then made several suggestions concerning the mold construction. The good relationship between this company and the vendor enabled the company to take advantage of rapid prototyping and resulted in significant savings in development time.

Sterilization and Shelf Life

If a device is to be sterilized prior to use, the sterilization method should be chosen early in the design cycle. Many tests (such as biocompatibility, fatigue testing, shelf life, etc.) require sterilized samples. In addition, the selection of materials and some aspects of the design and the selection of sterilization method are not independent events. Not all materials can withstand gamma radiation or the temperatures and moistures of steam autoclaving. The use of ethylene oxide gas or chemical sterilization requires a design that is accessible to the sterilizing agent.

Even though a company may offer the device nonsterile, the FDA has taken the position that instructions for use must include recommendations for proper cleaning and sterilization if required prior to use. If the customer is responsible for sterilizing the device, sterilization methods are limited. Most medical device users have access to autoclaving or gas sterilization. Some cold sterilization methods may be acceptable, but radiation sterilization is not generally available.

Once the sterilization method is chosen, it must be validated. Again, this is true even if the customer is responsible for sterilization. Most companies offering sterilization services will assist in the validation process. The number of samples required for validation will depend on the sterilization method chosen and the how well the product compares to other similar products. However the validation process may require 40 to 100 or more samples. Thus it is a good idea to save scrap product that could possibly be used for part of the validation study. Again, it is important to work with the sterilization vendor. Some contract labs will also assist in developing a validation plan.

Prototype samples and some scrap might also be useful in conducting shelf life studies. Product can be set aside to age and then tested to determine if any changes have occurred. Aging can be accelerated. It is generally accepted that every 8-10°C increase in temperature doubles reaction rates and thus doubles the rate of aging. Some contract labs will age samples in a temperature controlled chamber. Some protocols include aging at low and high humidity as well as a freezing cycle, which lends some additional credibility to the data. This data is generally acceptable in support of applications to regulatory agencies. However, devices should be set aside to confirm the accelerated aging results at a later date. Obviously, the sooner the samples are set aside, the sooner this data will be available.

Shelf life samples must represent the finished devices, including sterilization where applicable. Data should include the results of tests on aged devices demonstrating that the products meet their original specifications. Equivalent unaged samples should also be tested, unless data exists from previous testing. A statistical comparison of the data from aged and unaged samples demonstrates that the product's properties do not change significantly over time.

Although you use standard off-the-shelf packaging, you still must demonstrate that your packaging and sterilization methods result in a packaged product that will be sterile for the projected shelf life. This can be done by testing aged packaging. This testing includes demonstrating the product is sterile and that the package withstands a microbial challenge. Many contract labs have standard protocols for these tests.

A carefully written protocol for testing both the device and the packaging shelf life will minimize the number of samples required to meet these requirements. However, an early commitment to a sterilization method and to a packaging type is necessary to avoid lengthy post development testing.

Case History #7

The FDA audited a small company manufacturing a number of products, including metal instruments. Among other observations on the 483 form (a list of GMP violations issued by the Agency), was the claim that these products were mislabeled because labeling did not contain instructions for cleaning and sterilization. All of these products were sold nonsterile. However, the customer had to sterilize the instruments prior to use. The devices also had to be cleaned prior to reuse. In order to get their products back on the market, the company was forced to conduct cleaning and sterilization validation studies and modify their labeling. This was a major project, costing significant money and time.

Case History #8

A start-up company filed an Investigational Device Exemption for a feasibility study. Included among all of the data submitted were the results of a life cycle test. These results took several years to accumulate, because of the limited number of test stations and the time required to simulate 2-10 years of use. The reviewer noted that these tests should use samples as received by the customer, i.e., sterilized and aged. Since some of the samples had been sterilized and some had been stored before testing (waiting on the availability of a test station), the Agency accepted this data for the feasibility study. However, the company will have to repeat the test under more controlled conditions before applying for an IDE for an expanded clinical study.

Production Facilities

Decisions made early in the product development cycle have an effect on the production facility requirements. Some designs are amenable to automated assembly, while others require hand fabrication. Some processes require specialized equipment. Some materials and processes require temperature and humidity controls. Electronics may require protection from static discharge. As the design evolves, each change should be evaluated for its impact on future production needs.

If the special requirements are necessary, then these should be included in the facility plans. However, if these requirements do not contribute to the safety and efficacy of the device, their costs should be carefully examined.

There are several general factors to keep in mind in evaluating a process and laying out a facility:

1. Environmental control—the latest GMPs require suitable environmental control. This could include cleanliness, particulate control, static control, special lighting, etc. The level of cleanliness or particulate control required is up to the manufacturer. Of course, the rationale for these decisions must be documented. However, there are often industrial standards recognized as the norm for various types of devices. All environmental controls require monitoring and maintenance.

2. Adequate space—the space has to be adequate to prevent mix-ups. This can be done with suitably labeled areas and mobile carts. However, it is much easier if the process flows from incoming to finished product to warehousing. Particular attention must be paid to points in the process where processed product is not obviously different from unprocessed product (such as nonsterile and sterile packaged products). Label everything in the facility (either with a stick-on label or a processing record). Fabrication of commercial or clinical product must be separated from developmental or experimental product.

3. Equipment maintenance—All equipment must be maintained according to its specifications. Fixtures should be designed to facilitate this. Fixtures and equipment should have smooth surfaces for easy cleaning, access to parts likely to require replacement, and instruments that can be easily calibrated. All equipment must have a maintenance schedule (including cleaning). This can initially be based on engineering judgment. However, you will have to modify this schedule as maintenance related problems occur.

4. Instrument calibration—All instruments used to measure the product's properties or control the process need to be calibrated. Initially, instruments should be purchased with certificates of calibration. A calibration schedule can then be written, based on reasonable expectations of the instrument's ability to remain calibrated. A high precision caliper used in a critical operation may have to be calibrated daily. This could be done with several gage pins reserved for this purpose. However, a steel ruler may only require annual calibration. Use local metrology labs whenever possible. It may be possible to find companies specializing in weights or pressure gauges. Some of these companies will make house calls. If not, and the company is local, the instruments can be dropped off and picked up to minimize down time.

It should be noted that any facility or process requirements will have to be justified. Testing will be necessary to document that the facility or equipment is capable of meeting these requirements. The cost of the required maintenance and calibration programs will depend upon how precise and complicated the process must be. This should be kept in mind while designing the device. Steps should be taken to avoid unnecessary tolerances or process steps that can increase the cost of producing the device.

Case History #9

A start-up operation, whose objective was the development and commercialization of an implant, did all of the prototyping work (product and process) in a small laboratory. As work progressed toward commercialization, a production facility was leased and a floor plan developed. There were no moving parts or electronics that required a particular level of cleanliness. A review of the proposed process indicated that product could be kept in sealed containers and thus not be exposed to particulates for extended periods of time. As could best be ascertained, class 10,000 clean rooms were typically used in the manufacture of similar products. Therefore, it was decided to build a class 10,000 production facility. Incoming material would be cleaned prior to entering production and product packaged inside the clean room.

The only remaining environmental issue was the generation of static electricity during an operation involving dynamic contact between two dissimilar plastics. This static electricity attracted particles, even though the operation was done in the clean room. A deionizing air gun was installed at the point of contact to control this static.

Several pieces of used equipment were purchased for production. These were cleaned, rebuilt and painted, so that they would be easy to clean. The quantities that required measurement were time, temperature, and dimensions. The Naval Observatory time signal was used to calibrate a master stop watch. A calibrated thermometer was purchased (and later calibrated by an outside service). All micrometers, rulers, etc. were calibrated against certified gage blocks that were used only for this purpose. Any other calibration was done by outside services.

Product was fabricated at the extremes of the process tolerances and tested. The results were compared to the specifications, thus demonstrating that the process would produce devices within specification. Finally, these same results were compared to results obtained from competitive products, demonstrating that the facility produced state of the art devices.

Conclusion

Small size has advantages and disadvantages when it comes to developing medical devices. Regulatory agencies do not differentiate between small start-up operations and major international corporations. The ISO 9000 Quality Standard covers companies of all sizes[1]. Customers expect to get value and quality in a product, regardless of the size of the company making that product. Unfortunately, a small company lacks the resources (in personnel, equipment and capital) of a large company. This lack of resources can be a major disadvantage in developing and marketing a new device.

The major advantage of being small is the ability to communicate ideas and goals. Lines of communication are short in a small start-up company. There is less of a potential to miscommunicate information between people and departments in a small company. One of the major sources of delays and mistakes during product development occurs at the interfaces between departments. The new GMP (and the ISO 9000) regulations on design history are aimed at minimizing mistakes occurring due to lack of interdepartmental communication.[2] The effect of organizational size on the product development process is well documented. There are many horror stories resulting from the "throw it over the wall to manufacturing" syndrome. Large companies have tried skunk works, project teams, matrix organizations, reengineering and cross-function integration in order to regain the advantage of being a small company.[3,4]

Another advantage a small company could enjoy is the ability to focus on one goal. Often large companies are so involved in defending each of their market segments, refining old products and developing new devices, that their resources are diluted. If a start-up operation chooses to focus on one well-defined goal, it may actually be possible to bring more of certain resources to bear.

A successful small company takes advantage of its size and finds ways of overcoming the lack of resources. If you do not have a Quality Control or Regulatory function, then you must keep these needs in mind as you develop your idea. Use consultants if necessary. Attend seminars. Join local networking groups. Subscribe to trade journals. If you lack the tools or instruments to test your prototypes properly, find vendors with the necessary expertise. Use the Small Manufacturer's Assistance office of the FDA.

Remember that quality and ease-of-manufacturability are designed into a product. Both of these impact the future cost of producing a device. It is far easier, and less costly, to correct mistakes early in the design phase than it is late in the testing phase.

One sure fire method to seriously delay the commercialization of a product is to withdraw the device from a clinical study or initial market introduction to correct a problem that should have been discovered during the development phase. Not only is time lost in correcting the problem, but time is lost in convincing the investigators or customers that the problem has been solved.

A second method guaranteed to slow product development is to take each project requirement as it occurs. Plan for long lead items such as sterilization and shelf life testing, facility requirements, special testing for regulatory agency approvals, etc. Start these as soon as possible instead of waiting until all of the preceding tasks are completed.

Finally, document everything as you go along, in order to avoid unpleasant surprises down the road. Surprises usually cost time and money. Record, check, and organize the original specifications or plans, test methods, results and your rationale for product design decisions.

Obviously, none of these steps will eliminate the risk in a startup operation. However, these steps will help manage that risk and prevent you from repeating mistakes that others have made.

References

1. Johnson PL. ISO 9000—Meeting The New International Standards. New York, New York: McGraw-Hill, Inc., 1993.
2. Medical Device Quality Systems Manual, A Small Entity Compliance Guide; U.S. Department of Health and Human Services, FDA 97-4179, Dec. 1996.
3. Miller R. Applying Quality Practices to R&D; Research & Technology Management March-April 1995; 47-54.
4. Hammer M. Beyond Reengineering. New York, New York: Harper Collins Publishers, Inc. 1996.

Chapter 7

Tissue Engineering Constructs and Commercialization

Kelvin G.M. Brockbank

Tissue engineering is an interdisciplinary field that applies the principles of engineering (materials science and biomedical engineering) and the life sciences (biochemistry, genetics, cell and molecular biology) to the development of biological substitutes that can restore, maintain, or improve tissue functions. In its broader definition, tissue engineering includes isolated cells, tissue-inducing substances, and cells placed on or within matrices. However, in this instance the discussion of tissue engineering is limited to the development, design and implantation of devices consisting of matrices in association with cells, which can migrate, differenciate and perform normal cell/tissue functions. The matrices can be fashioned from natural materials such as collagen or from synthetic polymers. The cellular components may be of human or animal origin, with or without genetic modification. The purpose of this chapter is to present some of the key commercialization issues which exist in the new field of tissue engineering and consider how to utilize these as potential business opportunities.

The largest market for tissue engineered products is replacement of structurally or physiologically deficient or diseased tissues and organs in humans. The potential markets for tissue engineered products vary extremely both in size and degree of market development. For example, a recent report[1] indicated that the heart valve replacement and skin repair product markets have maximum potential market sizes of $225 and $5,945 million, respectively. Because the heart valve market is well developed, new products must compete with existing products for market share. In contrast, the skin market is virtually untapped, with room for many new products for a variety of clinical indications. Revenues in the total market are anticipated to grow at double-digit rates for the next five years,[1] making this a potentially rewarding field for investment. Tissue engineering may eventually address diseases and disorders which account for approximately half of current annual U.S. health care costs, which are estimated to be approximately one trillion dollars at this time.[2-5]

Tissue engineering companies are developing new generations of medical products not easily accommodated within traditional Food and Drug Administration classifications and definitions. Hybrid matrix/live cell-containing devices, which may have attributes of drugs or biologicals are seemingly subject to multiple regulatory definitions and classifications. Historically, the FDA has responded to the scientific and medical challenges presented by new technology by involving two or more FDA centers in product review with one FDA agency taking the primary responsibility. However, at the present time, products composed of or intended to contain intact cells fall within the jurisdiction of the Center for Biologics Evaluation and Research (CBER). It is extremely clear that hybrid products (in which the

Biomaterials in the Design and Reliability of Medical Devices, edited by Michael N. Helmus

primary mechanism of action is that of the somatic cell therapy component) will be regulated as biological products. It is not as clear whether products in which the matrix of the hybrid product is the major mechanism of action (such as in skin, heart valve or ligament constructs) will be devices or biologics. Both of the allogeneic hybrid skin graft products of Organogenesis, Inc., and Advanced Tissue Sciences, Inc., are being regulated as devices. The FDA and other concerned parties are working to formulate regulations and documents (such as points to consider and guidance documents) to clarify these issues. A list of some of the important historical regulatory milestones and more recent documents of relevance for tissue engineered products are listed in Table 7.1.

The first FDA approval of an engineered tissue product, without a living cellular component, occurred with the PreMarket Application (PMA) approval for Integra™ Artificial skin on March 1, 1996. More recently on May 22, 1998 Organogenesis received the first PMA approval for a hybrid product (Apligraf™) with living keratinocytes and fibroblasts for treatment of venous leg ulcers. Subsequently, on June 20, 2000, Apligraf™ was approved by the FDA for a second major application in the treatment of diabetic foot ulcers.

Systematic transplantation of living tissues and organs has become an every day event. Although there are significant benefits, there are also many problems associated with transplantation procedures. First, there is a significant shortage of donor organs. More than 10,000 people have died during the past 5 years while waiting for an organ transplant. Many patients must undergo expensive procedures, such as kidney dialysis, while on the transplant waiting list. Secondly, transmission of infectious agents, such as acquired immunodeficiency syndrome (AIDS) or hepatitis C, from donors to the transplant recipients are of concern. Furthermore, transplant recipients must remain on costly immunosuppressive agents for the remainder of their lives. The ultimate potential annual U.S. market size for organ and tissue transplants projected by Drs. Vacanti and Langer,[2] assuming an unlimited supply of transplants for all potential applications, is indicated Table 7.2. However, many scientific advances in the fields of tissue engineering and xenotransplantation must be made for this potential to materialize. The numbers are also predicated on transplantation being such a safe procedure that it would be considered appropriate therapy for a wide range of organ and tissue diseases for which transplantation would not presently be considered an option. The availability of tissue engineered products will change the way that medicine will be practiced in the future by providing more efficient lower cost alternatives to current tissue restoration and organ transplantation techniques.

Development of the full potential of tissue engineering is dependent upon major technological innovation. The National Institute of Standards recently identified some research areas in which substantial technical innovation is required (Table 7.3).[9] Discussion of all these opportunities for technical innovation and commercialization is beyond the intent of this chapter. The discussion is limited to two to illustrate the decision process used to determine whether or not a technical opportunity is also a wise business venture.

Footnote. Life Science Holdings, Inc., the parent company of Organ Recovery Systems, Inc., identified development of effective transport solutions and devices to enable product distribution and methods to increase product shelf life as commercial opportunities. Life Science Holdings had acquired rights to several technical innovations in the field of low temperature biology and following extensive due diligence, established Organ Recovery Systems to develop storage and transportation products. From a corporate perspective, considerable care must be taken prior to launching an all out product research and development effort.

Involvement in projects based on prior investment or an emotional attachment, "invented here" syndrome, is not adequate justification for further research and development. The product concepts considered were subjected to a series of tests, which are listed in Table 7.4, before committing to long-term research and development programs.

Table 7.1. Regulatory milestones and recent documents which impact engineered tissue products

Year	Milestone
1973	Federal Regulation: **General Biological Products** (21 CFR 610, 38 FR 32056)
1975	Federal Regulation: **Blood & Blood Components** (21 CFR 606, 40 FR 53532)
1978	Federal Regulations: **Finished Pharmaceuticals** (21 CFR 211, 43 FR 45077)
1993	Application of current authorities to human somatic cell therapy products (58 FR53248) "The relevant function of the cells, if known, and/or relevant products biosynthesized by the cells should be defined and quantitated as a measure of potency."
1993	Human tissue intended for transplantation. FDA indicates that transplantation falls within their jurisdiction and that they may regulate the industry at some future time (58 FR 65514)
1993	Animal cells and tissues as somatic therapy (58 FR 5324 10/14/93)
1996	Guidance on applications for products comprised of living autologous cells manipulated *ex vivo* and intended for structural repair of reconstruction (FR 04/26/96)
1998	Establishment registration and listing for manufacturers of human cell and tissue-based products (FR 05/14/98)
1998	Human tissue intended for transplantation. Regulation effective January 26, 1998 (FR 06/29/98
1999	Suitability determination for donors of Human cellular and tissue-based products. (FR 09/30-99)

*For a full listing of relevant documents and copies call the Center for Biologics Evaluation and Research on (800) 835-4709.

Table 7.2. Potential U.S. organ & tissue markets

Structure	Procedures/Year
Skin	4,750,000
Cartilage	1,132,100
Blood Vessels	1,100,000
Pancreas	728,000
Kidney	600,000
Breast	261,000
Liver	155,000
Tendon & Ligament	123,000
Intestine	100,000
Ureter & Urethra	81,900
Heart Valves	65,000
Bladder	57,200

Material modified from references 2, 5

Table 7.3. Opportunities for commercialization

Biomaterials	Cellular components
· Naturally-derived, synthetic or hybrid materials · Permissive of cellular activities · Minimal host reactivity · Desirable physical and chemical features	· Large scale cell culture methods · Sources, such as transgenic animals · Modulation of cell functions genetically or environmentally · Avoidance of recipient immune response
Manufacturing processes	**Implantation technologies**
· Automation and scale up · Sterilization · Product storage · Transportation of product	· Devices to aid in transplantation · Methods for monitoring transplant procedures · Tests to follow functional and structural integration

Table 7.4. General criteria for product development

- Prospectively fulfills unmet need in potentially large markets
- Shows strong likelihood of technical feasibility, efficacy and cost effectiveness
- Unique to the market or first in market with strong proprietary position
- Time to market less than five years
- Cost to market within financial means of the Company and its partners without undue risk

Case Studies: Development of Effective Transport Solutions and Devices to Enable Product Distribution

The first anticipated products being developed by the Company are temperature controlled shipping units with data logging capabilities. These devices will be used for refrigerated transportation of highly perishable medical products such as stem cells, organs for transplantation and tissue engineered living replacement parts. The first organ transportation device has kidney perfusion capabilities. This organ transport device, in combination with effective organ preservation solutions, should result in more human organs (kidneys, livers, and hearts) being available for transplantation by expansion of the acceptable postmortem organ ischemia time for organ acceptance. This device will also be effective for transport of xenogeneic organs when they are approved for human use. These devices are being developed to meet the following design criteria:

- Compact, light weight, and strong
- High technology insulation, which reduces coolant requirements
- Simple, reliable, and not requiring continuous attention
- Monitoring, documentation, and feedback control capabilities

Current model devices for organ transport can maintain temperatures for 2 days. Future devices will maintain temperature for longer periods and enable organs and tissue engineered products to be distributed world wide. At the present time, a kidney transport device (Fig. 7.1) and a chemically defined solution (Unisol^{TM}) designed to maintain cell viability and tissue functions during refrigerated transportation are in preclinical trials.

How do these products hold up by our general criteria for product development (Table 7.4)? According to our internal confidential review, these products demonstrated a strong likelihood

Table 7.5. Potential U.S. customers for storage and transportation products

Company	Engineered Products
Advanced Tissue Sciences, Inc.	Skin, articular cartilage, menisci, heart valves
Amphioxus Inc.	Artificial liver
Baxter Healthcare Corporation	Skin, cartilage, heart valves and blood vessels
BioHybrid Technologies, Inc.	Encapsulated tissues
CarboMedics, Inc.	Heart valves
CellCo	Research products for tissue engineering
Cellex Biosciences, Inc.	Artificial liver
Cell Genesys, Inc.	Universal cell transplant products
Circe Biomedical	Pancreas and liver
Clonetics, Inc.	Research products for tissue engineering
CryoLife, Inc.	Heart valves and ligaments
Genzyme Tissue Repair	Articular cartilage and skin
Hepatix, Inc.	Artificial liver
Integra LifeSciences Corporation	Skin, cartilage, musculoskeletal tissues and organs
LifeCell Corporation	Skin, heart valves and vascular grafts
Life Technologies, Inc.	Research products for tissue engineering
Medtronic, Inc.	Heart valves
National Disease Research Interchange	Research products for tissue engineering
Organogenesis, Inc.	Skin, liver and vascular grafts
Ortec International, Inc.	Skin
Progenitor, Inc.	Genetically engineered "mini-organs"
Reprogenesis, Inc.	Ureters, bladders, and breasts
SoloHill Labs, Inc.	Encapsulated tissues
St. Jude Medical, Inc.	Heart valves
Synergy Research Corporation	Encapsulated tissues
Tissue engineering, Inc.	Vascular grafts, ligaments, tendons, Periodontal tissues and glands
VivoRx, Inc.	Encapsulated pancreatic islets

of technical feasibility, efficacy and cost effectiveness. They are also expected to be unique to the market or first in the market and are protected by a very strong proprietary position due to the Company's aggressive pursuit of patents and technology licensing. The time to market should be less than five years because regulatory hurdles are relatively low and much of the hardware is available off the shelf. These products not only prospectively fulfill an unmet need in potentially large markets (namely the entire field of tissue engineered biological products and xenogeneic organs), but also have more immediate markets for shipment of highly perishable biomedical materials such as stem cells and organ transplants. Finally, the Company determined that these projects were within current financial means and identified strategies for future funding based upon achievement of specific project milestones.

Development of Methods to Increase Product Shelf-life

The product development criteria (Table 7.4.) for product shelf life methods were also reviewed at great length by Organ Recovery Systems. There was no question regarding the

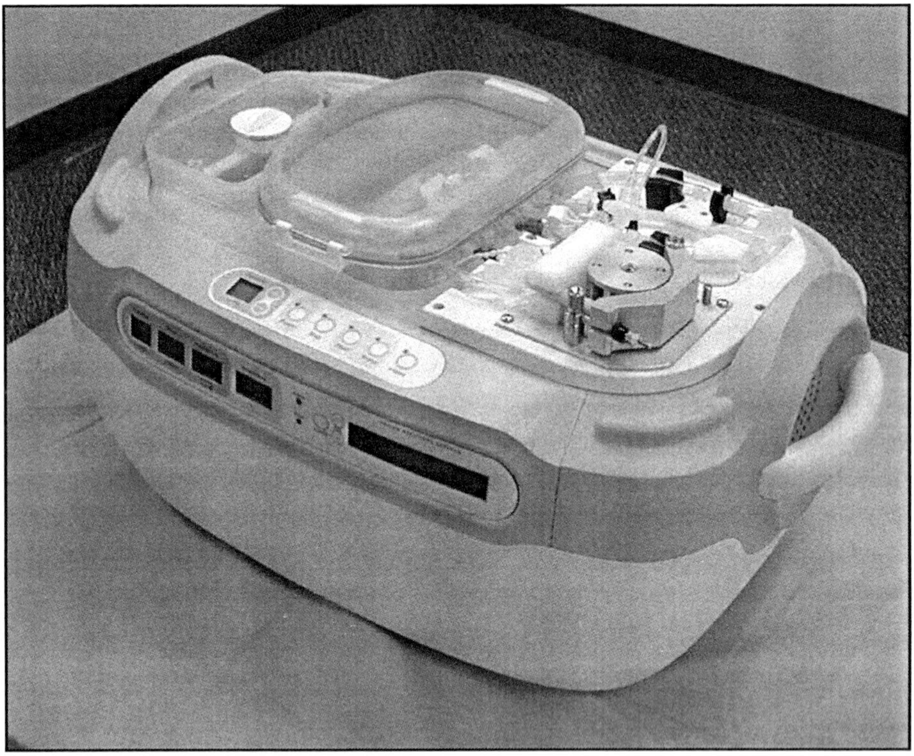

Fig. 7.1. Kidney transport device previewed at the International Transplantation Society meeting in Rome, Italy (August 2000). This device is not available for human use.

opportunity to fill unmet needs in potentially large markets. Such methods were considered to be technically feasible and could be designed to be both efficacious and relatively cost effective. The technology would be both unique to the market and probably first in the market with a very strong proprietary position based upon multiple patent families and trade secrets. The only methods currently used for unlimited storage and stabilization of cells and tissues involve the application of cryobiology.[6-8] These methods are generally limited in application to single cells and simple cell aggregates. The technical barriers associated with ice formation and cryoprotectant toxicity have blocked progress in the extension of cryobiology methods to larger biological structures. The first barrier (ice formation) is significant; however, the later is largely an engineering issue. Ice may form and cause problems for cell and tissue stabilization and storage intracellularly and extracellularly, both within the tissue matrix and around the biological materials. The Company has two innovative approaches to defeating the technical barrier presented by ice.

The first approach is to control ice formation in such a manner that the ice which forms does not have opportunities to grow in forms which cause either cellular or matrix damage. Ice control will be achieved by combining proprietary synthetic ice blockers with traditional cryoprotectants. Synthetic ice blocking molecules are being designed to bond with ice crystals. Some of these compounds have turned out to be available "off-the-shelf," but have **not** been identified previously as having antifreeze potential; others are presently being synthesized.

The second approach is complete avoidance of ice formation by vitrification. Using this approach, a noncrystalline solid structure (glass) is achieved by replacing at least 50% of the water with cryoprotective chemicals. The major barrier to development of vitrification solution formulations is screening the vast quantity of potential cryoprotective chemicals, combinations and concentrations that are possible. The technical barriers are achievable engineering issues relating to addition and removal of a high concentration of cryoprotective agents in such a manner that toxicity is avoided and effective warming techniques are perfected. These technical barriers should be easier to overcome for tissue engineered structures once optimal vitrification solutions have been developed.[9,10]

Unfortunately, continuing our review of criteria from Table 7.4, the time to market for most applications in tissue engineering for new storage technology is probably greater than five years and the cost to market was not considered to be without undue financial risk by the Company and its partners. This resulted in the development of new storage methods for tissue engineered products being given a low priority. This decision was subsequently reversed when funding was obtained in response to a request for proposals from the National Institute of Standards & Technology (NIST).[11] The funding obtained from NIST reduced the financial risks of this research program for the Company. At this time the development of molecular approaches to ice control for engineered tissue storage has the highest corporate priority.

Ultimately, the success of tissue engineered products, in common with any highly perishable product, depends upon the availability of practical product storage and transportation methods. The customers for the Company's storage and transportation products will be tissue engineering organizations, organ procurement organizations, hospitals, tissue processing and banking organizations and companies which supply reagents and biological materials to research organizations pursuing tissue engineering programs (A partial list of potential corporate customers is given in Table 7.5).

In conclusion, the field of tissue engineering presents both challenges and opportunities for the development of new medical products but great care should be taken in review of potential opportunities before committing to product development.

References

1. U.S. Organ Transplant and Related Product Markets, Frost & Sullivan, 1996.
2. Langer R, Vacanti JP. Tissue Engineering. Science 1993; 260:920.
3. Nerem RM, Sambaris A. Tissue Engineering. 1995; 1:3.
4. Wilkerson Group, Inc., Research on Market Potential for Tissue Engineering, 1992.
5. Heart and Stroke Facts—1996 Statistical Supplement. American Heart Association.
6. Mazur P. Freezing of living cells: Mechanisms and implications. Am J Physiol 1984; 247:125.
7. Karow AM. Biophysical and chemical considerations in cryopreservation. In: Karow AM, Pegg DE, eds. Organ preservation for transplantation. New York: Dekker 1981:113.
8. Brockbank KGM. Essentials of Cryobiology. In: KGM Brockbank, ed. Principles of Autologous, Allogeneic, and Cryopreserved Venous Transplantation. Austin, TX: R.G. Landes Company, (Medical Intelligence Unit Series) and Springer-Verlag, 1995.
9. Song YC, Khirabadi BS, Lightfoor FG et al. Avoidance of ice by vitreous cryopreservation dramatically improves the function of vascular grafts. Nature Biotechnology 2000; 18:296-299.
10. Brockbank KGM, Lightfoot FG, Song YC et al. Interstitial ice formation in cryopreserved homografts: A possible cause of tissue deterioration and calcification in vivo. J Heart Valve Dis 2000; 9:200-206.
11. Request for Proposals for the ATP Focused Program Competition 97-07, National Institute of Standards and Technology, February 1997.

Chapter 8

Testing of Biomaterials Modified with Bioactive Molecules: A Case Study

Katherine S. Tweden

The majority of medical devices available today are manufactured of relatively inert materials to discourage aggressive biological responses. It has become clear in the last decade or more that the success of traditional materials in many medical devices is unsatisfactory. Specifically, the recipients of state-of-the-art mechanical heart valves still require life long anticoagulation therapy,[17] small diameter (< 6 mm ID) synthetic vascular prostheses fail due to thrombosis or intimal hyperplasia,[2] biosensors work only temporarily because of biofouling, and hip prostheses and dental implants loosen with time because of poor interaction with the surrounding tissue.[11] However, the economic and legal hurdles to developing new materials are overwhelming for most companies especially in the face of supplier giants such as DuPont pulling out of the field for long term implantation such well studied materials as Dacron® polyester and Teflon®. These problems have led medical researchers to concentrate their efforts on improving existing materials using surface modification. Ideally, the inherent physical properties of the material are not changed by the modification process.

Two approaches have been taken for optimizing the biologic response of materials using surface modification. The first approach has been to mask the materials with coatings that render them passive or relatively nonadhesive biologically. This approach has been used in applications in which biological deposition needs to be minimal such as vascular catheters, biosensors and other cardiovascular devices. The focus in this approach has been coatings such as fluoropolymers, polyethylene oxide, polyacrylamide, polyvinylpyrolidone, albumin, pyrolytic carbons and silanes because of their promise for the prevention of an aggressive biological response.[13,15,20,70] The success of these passivating coatings has been variable. In fact, recent reanalysis of the platelet response to pyrolytic carbons with state-of-the-art instrumentation has revealed that platelets have an aggressive response to carbons rather than a passive one as was originally thought.[23]

The second approach to making existing materials more acceptable biologically has been to modify them with bioactive molecules that allow them to actively participate in the biological interaction. For example, many have studied ways to promote endothelialization of materials used in cardiovascular devices since healthy, functional endothelium provides a physiologic, nonthrombogenic, and infection-resistant surface. Modification with cell adhesion molecules (CAMs) and growth factors (GFs) that promote the attachment and growth of this cell type has been the strategy for encouraging endothelialization of materials.[19,25,35,36]

Biomaterials in the Design and Reliability of Medical Devices, edited by Michael N. Helmus

The CAMs, GFs, and other molecules studied for this purpose include arginine-glutamic acid-aspartic acid-valine (REDV)—and arginine-glycine-aspartic acid (RGD)—containing peptides, fibronectin, laminin, heparin, fibrin glue, and fibroblast growth factors. Potentially, any biologically active molecule can be immobilized on material surfaces if the immobilization process is adequately gentle. Whether or not the molecule retains its biological activity needs to be demonstrated on a case-by-case basis. The biologically active molecules that are generating the most interest for surface modification include cell adhesion molecules, antithrombotic/thrombolytic/antiplatelet agents, growth factors, and antimicrobials.[15,27,37,42,83]

In contrast to surface modification, traditional materials have also been used as delivery vehicles to deliver drugs to effect the biological response to the device. For example, heparin was shown to minimize thrombus formation associated with mechanical heart valves when delivered from the valve sewing cuff.[69] Basic fibroblast growth factor has also been delivered from expanded polytetrafluoroethylene (ePTFE) vacular prostheses to promote healing.[82] Work has also been done on the delivery of anticalcification agents for the prevention of bioprosthetic tissue valve calcification (Hirsch et al, 1993). For a thorough discussion on the differences between bound versus releasable agents see Hubbell (1993). There are also bulk materials that are considered bioactive such as bioglass, calcium phosphates, and collagens. Some groups have synthesized polymers with bioactive groups such as ProNectin™ F which is a genetically engineered silk-like protein polymer incorporating multiple copies of the RGD cell adhesion peptide.[9] In addition, with the ongoing interest in heparin as an antithrombotic agent others have reported on new block copolymers that contain heparin.[80]

To bring medical devices composed of materials modified with bioactive molecules to market, the bioactive material has to be able to withstand a manufacturing environment which includes assembly, sterilization and long term storage before and after assembly (shelf life). This chapter addresses methods that can be used to characterize materials modified with bioactive molecules to determine their appropriateness for use in medical devices. Specifically, methods for characterization of the nature and uniformity, quantitation, assessment of the biological activity *in vitro* and in vivo, and determination of manufacturing ruggedness of the suface modified materials are discussed. See Table 1 for an outline of the techniques discussed below. Following this section, the testing that was done to show bioactivity of textiles modified with a cell adhesion peptide for use in cardiovascular devices is discussed. With bulk bioactive materials the testing rationale discussed below should be followed in addition to appropriate physical and mechanical testing to ensure that these properties meet the needs of the device. In addition, as discussed above there is much activity in the development of devices that incorporate controlled release of biologically active molecules in their design. The characterization of this important class of device will not be addressed in this chapter. Methods of surface modification will also not be addressed. A summary on this topic can be found in Hoffman (1987) and Sefton et al (1987). The terms coating and modification are used interchangeably.

Characterization of the Nature and Uniformity of the Modification

Once the bioactive substance of interest has been immobilized or coated on the substrate using, for example, either covalent coupling,[37] physical adsorption,[78] plasma polymerization,[83] ion-beam assisted deposition of metals,[72] or photochemical methods,[15] the nature of the modification can be assessed using chemical and surface energetic methods. The information obtained can be used to correlate the surface chemistry with the biologic response to the material and to demonstrate control over the modification process. It is also of interest to assess the uniformity of the modification to ensure that there will be a relatively uniform biological response to the material.

Table 8.1. Characterization of bioactive materials

Chemical Nature/ Energetics	Morphology	Uniformity	Quantitation	In vitro Bioactivity	In vivo Bioactivity	Manufacturability
ATR-IR[a]	SEM	SEM/colloidal Au	radiolabeling	CAMs[f] -cell adhesion, spreading -focal contacts -matrix prod.	Nonfunctional -vascular patch -subdermal -intramuscular -intraperitoneal -intramedullary	handling
XPS[b]	AFM/SFM[e]	immunoassay	fluorescence	GF[g] -cell prolif. -chemotaxis -matrix prod.	Functional -final device config. in appropriate model	sterilization
ISS[c]	profilometry	autoradiography	immunoassay	AT[h] -platelet act. -coagulation cascade effects -etc.		shelf life
SIMS[d]			colorimetric	AM[i] -adhesion -inhibition zone		
AES[j]			chromatography			
Contact angle			spectroscopy			

a ATR-IR = attenuated total reflectance-infrared spectroscopy, b XPS = x-ray photoelectron spectroscopy, c ISS = ion scattering spectroscopy, d SIMs = secondary ion mass spectroscopy, e AFM/SFM = atomic/scanning force microscopy, f CAMs = cell adhesion molecules, g GF = growth factors, h AT = antithrombotics, i AM = antimicrobials, j AES = auger electron spectroscopy.

Techniques that are used to chemically characterize surface modified materials include attenuated total reflectance infrared spectroscopy (ATR-IR),[83] X-ray photoelectron spectroscopy (XPS),[83] secondary ion mass spectroscopy (SIMs, static or time-of-flight, for polymer surfaces,), ion scattering spectroscopy (ISS)[63] and auger electron spectroscopy (AES, for materials other than polymers).[63] See Ratner (1982) for the discussion of additional techniques. Any changes to the morphology or topography of the surface can typically be assessed using scanning electron microscopy (SEM), profilometry (stylus technique)[63] or atomic or scanning force microscopy (AFM, SFM).[37] Many biological molecules can also be labelled with colloidal gold and imaged using SEM.[24] Surface energetics can be determined using contact angle analysis.[85] Solid phase immunoassays can be used to determine the uniformity and density of molecules to which antibodies can be raised.[44,71] Autoradiography is a simple way to assess uniformity of radiolabelled materials.

With ATR-infrared spectroscopy the surface modification has to represent at least 5 weight percent of the surface mass in order to get an adequate signal. The absorption of infrared radiation causes characteristic vibrations in materials which are used to construct a spectrum that can be used to determine chemical nature and molecular structure. The infrared beam samples quite deeply (1-5 μm) so depending on the coating thickness, the underlying substrate may also be sampled.[28] However, ATR-IR can prove to be a valuable, inexpensive way to characterize the chemical composition of many modifications.

XPS or ESCA (electron spectroscopy for chemical analysis) is a nondestructive technique used to determine the composition of the outermost atomic layers (average depth of penetration is 30 Å) of a material by analyzing the photoelectrons emitted from the x-ray flooded sample. All elements can be detected, with the exception of hydrogen, with a detectability limit of 0.05 atom percent. Chemical depth profiling can also be done with the use of an inert gas sputter ion gun. This technique is especially useful if the coating has different atomic species than the substrate (for example, an amino acid coating on a hydrocarbon can be seen with XPS by the occurrence of a N peak). Static SIMS is a complimentary technique to XPS for qualitatively studying the outermost chemical structure of a solid through the analysis of whole molecular fragments removed by bombarding the sample with a low dose of ions (Ratner, 1982). AES is useful for determining the chemical composition of the top 50 Å of nonpolymeric material surfaces. This technique consists of bombarding samples with electrons and characterizing ejected auger electrons.[63]

Scanning electron microscopic analysis of the substrate before and after modification can be useful for obtaining direct information on the effect of the modification process on the topography of the substrate and/or for imaging the coating. AFM is an extremely sensitive method useful for assessing the three-dimensional structure or morphology of the surface. Under optimal conditions, this technique can resolve detail down to the atomic level.[52] AFM images are generated by monitoring the Z-movement of a cantilever with an attached probe tip that is scanned across the sample surface. Typical x-y scan sizes range from 10 by 10 nm to 10 by 10 μm and information such as mean root mean square (rms) roughness and z-range values (lowest to highest points) can be obtained. Some prefer to combine AFM or SFM information with low voltage, high resolution SEM (capable of macromolecular resolution) to ensure that there are no misinterpretations as to the true nature of the modification.[18] It is usually best to use a multi-technique approach to fully characterize a surface modified device.

Solid-phase immunoassays are useful for characterizing the uniformity of modifications when antibodies can be raised to the modifying molecule. Substances such as proteins and polysaccharides can stimulate an antibody response if seen as foreign from the host. Obviously it would not be wise to render a material strongly immunogenic. However, peptides and oligosaccharides which are more commonly used in surface modification can be conjugated to the immunogenic substrate keyhole limpet hemocyanin (KLH) to stimulate an antibody response for purposes of tracing the molecule.[29] Others have biotinylated surfaces and taken advantage of the high affinity avidin-biotin binding complex and the availability of biotinylated antibodies to image surfaces.[4] The antibodies can be labelled with fluorescent probes, enzymes for reaction with precipitating colorimetric substrates, or even gold labels for imaging. Coating uniformity can also be evaluated using autoradiography methods which consist of exposing materials with radiolabelled coatings to film at low temperatures (usually at -70°C) for various periods and result in an image of the coating.

Surface energy measurements obtained using contact angle analysis can provide empirical information on how the modification changed the energy and wettability of the surface. This method is sensitive to the very outermost atomic species (top 5 Å of the modification).[59] This technique, when combined with others, can be useful for elucidating the orientation of immobilized molecules.[59,60] Some groups use this technique as a quick assessment of the uniformity or completeness of the modification.[15]

Quantitation of the Modification

The amount of coating should be quantitated to determine the optimal amount of coating needed for biological effectiveness and to determine the effect of various challenges on the coating. Radiolabelling is one of the most commonly used methods to quantitate coatings.[37] Nonradioactive quantitation techniques include immunochemical assays, spectroscopy methods, chromatography (if the substance can be reliably stripped from the substrate or if the substrate can be hydrolyzed), fluorescent methods and colorimetric assays. With solid-phase immunoassays, appropriate controls are needed to ensure that background absorption is not an issue. Immunochemical assays are adaptable and can be used for the determination of the amount of coating on substrates by using a soluble substrate (such as orthophenylenediamine dihydrochloride).

Labelling molecules with fluorescent probes is an effective way to trace and quantitate modifications. The general classes of functional groups that can be modified are thiols, amines, aldehydes, ketones and carboxylic acids.[30] Fluorescein isothiocyanate (FITC) is probably the most commonly used fluorescent derivitization reagent. Specific proteins that have been labeled with FITC include actin and epidermal growth factor.[53,84]

ATR-IR spectroscopy can be used to quantitate the amount of coating by using a series of references with known concentrations. It is also useful to look at the density of a coating by IR by monitoring the ratio of a unique band in the coating with one in the substrate.[14]

Colorimetric assays have been used for quantitation of many molecules, for example, heparin immobilized on surfaces can be quantitated using the metachromatic dye toluidine blue (Smith et al, 1980). In addition, the amount of immobilized glucose oxidase (for detection of glucose) can be quantitated using an o-dianisidine activity assay.[12] The chemistry of many molecules can be exploited to quantitate their amount on modified biomaterials.

Assessment of the Biological Activity In Vitro

The biological activity of the molecule after immobilization cannot be assumed, it must be proven. For example, work with heparin immobilization in the past showed that a spacer molecule and end point attachment was necessary to fully preserve the anticoagulant activity of heparin.[16,41] The bioassay should assess the biological activities of most importance, for example CAMs should be tested at a minimum in a cell adhesion assay. It would also be of interest to assess the occurrence of cell spreading and focal attachments with this type of molecule.

Cell adhesion can be quantitated using colorimetric, fluorescent, or radioisotope assays. A typical assay would consist of incubating the cells with either a dye or fluorescent or radioisotope probe, solubilizing the dyed cells with a detergent such as sodium dodecyl sulfate (SDS) and assaying the level of probe released spectrophotometrically as compared to that released from a set of references. For example, one group has developed techniques to covalently label cells with FITC under physiologic conditions. The cells were lysed with detergent and the released fluorochrome was assessed quantitatively with a fluorescence spectrophotometer (Lewinsohn et al, 1988). This same group showed that cell number determination using a fluorometric approach was comparable to that obtained with ^{51}Cr-labelled cells. Another group has reported on labelling vascular cells with low concentrations of fluorescent carbiocyanine dyes without adversely affecting their proliferative capacity. It is suggested that this technique is applicable to tissue culture assays and perhaps cell detection in vivo.[62] Colorimetric probes that have been used for cell quantitation include toluidine blue and crystal violet.[15] Cell spreading can be imaged with fluorescence, scanning electron, or phase contrast microscopic techniques.

The presence of focal contacts are used to assess the quality of the adhesion of cells to materials modified with cell adhesion molecules. These focal contacts are an extracellular terminus of intracellular actin stress fibers.[7] Techniques that can be used to optically image these contacts are interference reflection microscopy (IRM)[21] and total internal reflection fluorescence microscopy (TIRFM).[1] These techniques are limited to materials that can be preadsorbed onto optical plates. Others have shown the presence of focal contacts using fluorescently labelled antibodies to talin.[38]

Changes in the cytotoxicity of a material as a result of surface modification (specifically to indicate a decrease in cytotoxicity) can be assessed using extract dilution assay (MEM elution) and agar diffusion assay.[56] In addition, another group reported on the use of fluorescein diacetate and ethidium bromide as fluorescent probes to discriminate between intact and membrane-damaged cells, respectively.[61] Surface modified materials for cardiovascular applications should also be assessed for changes in blood compatibility and microbe adhesion, especially for CAM and GF modifications.[26]

The anticoagulant properties of antithrombotics should be assessed using specific assays such as the inhibition of factor Xa for heparin[83] in addition to more global tests such as activated partial thromboplastin time (APTT), and prothrombin time (PT). Demonstration of nonthrombogenicity of modified materials has been done using platelet assays and arteriovenous shunt studies.[39,75] Many books and chapters have been devoted to the testing of the blood compatibility of materials. Clearly many of the techniques discussed in these references would be appropriate for materials modified with antithrombotics.[46,66]

Immobilized antimicrobials should be assayed for their ability to kill or inhibit the microbe that is most problematic in the site the device will be placed.[42] Tests for efficacy include adherence experiments (determine if bacteria will adhere to the treated material), zone of inhibition assays and determination of the minimum inhibitory concentration.

Growth factors are potent mitogens of specific cells, so they should be assayed for their ability to stimulate cellular proliferation after immobilization. Other biological activities stimulated by growth factors include chemotaxis, cell differentiation, and extracellular matrix production. The activities demonstrated by the soluble growth factor should still be present in an immobilized factor.[6,40] Osteopontin is an interesting molecule that has been proposed for the enhancement of hard tissue integration of devices due to its cell adhesion and growth factor activities (O'Neal et al, 1992). Platelet-derived growth factor has been shown to influence the orientation of cells on titanium alloy discs for dental implant applications.[50]

The effect of the surface modification on the function of appropriate cell types (for molecules other than growth factors) can demonstrate the benefits of a modification. For example, for cardiovascular bioactive materials designed to promote endothelialization it would be revealing to assess if endothelial cells cultured with the material have the ability to produce prostacyclin, an indication of their ability to express an anticoagulant phenotype. If chemotaxis is an important biological activity of the surface, it can be addressed using a modified Boyden chamber.[38] In this assay cells are stimulated to move through 8 μm pores towards the chemoattractant. Similarly, modifying half of the surface and assaying for the attraction of cells towards the modified part of the surface can address cell movement activities.[78]

In Vitro Challenges

Once the biological activity of the modified material is confirmed under ideal conditions (with an intact, unchallenged coating), these results should be compared with those obtained from modified materials challenged with environments that will be encountered in vivo, for example, to shear conditions of typical vascular grafts or prosthetic heart valves. These flow experiments can be done in saline as a more gentle test followed by plasma to determine if the coating can withstand the detergent effects of plasma. Some have used a rotating disc system to determine the effect of shear on coating integrity. In this system the coating is subjected to many levels of shear in one experiment (from zero at the center of the disc to the maximum at the edge of the disc, the magnitude of which is determined by the rotational velocity and the radius of the disc).[34,77]

Kottke-Marchant et al[45] reported on an in vitro model for the assessment of blood compatibility of vascular grafts that consists of simultaneously exposing a control silicone rubber circuit and a test silicone circuit that contains the vascular graft to anticoagulated human whole blood. The types of analysis done included cell counts, platelet release measurement, platelet aggregation, APTT, PT and scanning electron microscopy. Others have designed models that simulate left ventricular function to assess the in vitro performance and thrombogenicity of prosthetic heart valves.[24]

After each of these challenges, the integrity, bioactivity, and amount of bioactive molecule remaining should be assessed using the scheme discussed above. Biological deposition on material exposed to tissue fluids can be evaluated using techniques such as electron microscopy and perhaps ATR-IR spectroscopy.

Manufacturing Ruggedness

From a manufacturing point of view, of equal importance to showing the ability to modify a material with a biologically active coating is the ability of the modified material to withstand fabrication into a medical device, sterilization and long-term storage (shelf life). Fabrication of the bioactive material into the device typically requires extensive handling with forceps and gloved hands so a coating that easily scratches or rubs off is unacceptable unless it can be shown that the remaining biological activity of the material is adequate.

Ideally, the modified material must also be able to be sterilized after assembly into a device (there is typically more confidence in the sterility of a terminally sterilized device, although aseptic assembly is an option). The most common methods of sterilization for synthetics are steam, ethylene oxide (EtO) gas, and ionizing radiation (gamma rays, accelerated electrons). For tissue products the most common method is a mixture of alcohol and aldehydes. Other less commonly used modes of sterilization include plasma gas, peroxygen compounds (hydrogen peroxide, peracetic acid), propylene oxide, and halides in alcohol.[5]

Bioactive molecules such as antithrombotics and various growth factors typically cannot withstand steam or radiation sterilization, groups have tried less aggressive methods such as EtO or plasma gas. With heparin modified devices, EtO has been shown to decrease the biological activity of the material (data not shown, St. Jude Medical, Inc.). The majority of groups reporting studies in which sterile bioactive devices were tested (e.g., in cell culture systems) addressed sterilization by exposing samples to ultraviolet light (UV). However, UV will not penetrate most substances so it is effective in inactivation of surface bound organisms only. Clearly, this mode of sterilization is not adequate for most, if not all medical devices.

Finally, once the device is successfully assembled and sterilized using the bioactive material, it must be determined if the device has a reasonable shelf life. Minimum acceptable shelf lives are 4-5 years duration. Manufacturers do testing in real time and in accelerated conditions of high temperature and high humidity (simulating the device sitting on the loading dock in a tropical environment). After these challenges, it would be advised to assay for the quantity of coating remaining and the biological activity using some of the assays discussed above.

Assessment of the Biological Activity In Vivo

Assessment of the in vivo biological activity of the bioactive material can proceed in two phases; nonfunctional testing in which the material is subjected to the physiological milieu but not put into full function and, if this testing is successful, testing of the material in a final device configuration. An example of nonfunctional testing is using a vascular patch model to assess the healing and thrombotic response to a modified textile for a cardiovascular device application.[79] In addition, small animal models such as the rat or rabbit subcutaneous, intramuscular, and intraperitoneal models have been used to quickly and inexpensively assess soft tissue response to bioactive materials.[10] One group reported on the use of the rabbit subcutaneous model to assess the infection-resistance of a textile surface modified with an antibiotic. This model involved inoculating a modified textile sample with an appropriate microbe, implanting the sample in the dorsal subcutaneous tissue of a rabbit, and assessing the degree of infection and extent of tissue ingrowth present after one week post-implantation. To quickly determine the calcific potential of surface modified biologic tissue, the weanling rat subdermal model is preferred.[48] Hard tissue nonfunctional models include analyzing plugs of the biomaterial placed in long cortical bones such as the humerus or femur.[55] These nonfunctional tests are good, economical ways to screen the in vivo response of many bioactive materials. The enhancement of hard tissue wound healing using bioactive molecule coated substrates are typically tested in nonhealing hard tissue defects such as the primate calvarial defects.[64]

Based on the results of simple in vivo testing then only the most promising bioactive materials are tested in the relatively expensive final device configuration. It is appropriate to choose an animal model that has already been developed if it can be demonstrated using that model that the device fabricated with bioactive materials effects a different biologic response (hopefully improved) than the established control device. For example, the sheep valve replacement model is typically used for the testing of new prosthetic heart valve designs. However, if an improvement in blood compatibility is expected with a surface modification, the sheep has proven to be unsatisfactory because of the difference in the hemostatic systems between sheep and humans. In response to this deficiency, groups are determining the feasibility of the use of a pig valve replacement model since the pig hemostatic system is closer to humans than other nonprimates (Personal communication, Richard Bianco, Director of Cardiovascular Research Laboratory, U. of Minnesota). Vascular grafts are tested in the dog model primarily, but the sheep, pig, and primate model have been used also.[8]

Careful thought should be put into the type of evaluation that will be performed on the bioactive device in vivo. For example, Walenga[81] has performed studies in humans with the Jarvik-7-70 total artificial heart that indicated that an imbalance between the coagulation and fibrinolytic systems (as measured by plasma and cellular activation markers of these systems) was predictive of thrombotic events, in cases where the coagulation and platelet systems were highly activated, and bleeding events, in cases where the fibrinolytic system was highly activated. These same types of relatively noninvasive studies could be done in animal models for the assessment of the blood compatibility of cardiovascular devices if adequate cross reactivity of the antibodies used for the immunochemical studies can be demonstrated or by producing antibodies for the model animal antigens. For a review of other techniques used in hemocompatibility assessment see Sawyer et al.

Total hip joint replacement and fraction fixation devices have been tested in rats, cats, dogs, sheep and goats.[3] Dental implants are tested in dogs, sheep, primates, pigs, and rabbits. Good reviews of osteocompatibility and odontocompatibility assessment are found in Tencer et al[76] and Natiella.[54]

As in all experimentation, controls are critical in the testing of these devices. Animal-to-animal variability that confounds comparisons can be accounted for if the device can be configured so that the control and treated portions are part of the same device. For example, a vascular graft could be fabricated from half untreated and half treated fabric. Even so, large numbers of replicates are needed to determine if a statistically significant difference exists between the biological response to the unmodified component and the modified component. The number of replicates needed is dependent upon the type of data collected to assess the biological activity. Smaller sample sizes will be needed if the values of variables are expressed in the interval or ratio scales rather than reducing data to categories or success versus failure measurements. For example, if a device is modified with an antithrombotic agent and the level of thrombus is assessed by percent surface coverage or ranking, larger numbers of replicates will be needed for this analysis as compared to data such as the measure of tensile strength measurements of an explanted bone plate or the quantitation of markers of activation of the hemostatic system after implantation of a cardiovascular device.[51]

A thorough pathologic analysis of the explants is essential and should include gross and histological workup at a minimum. Electron microscopy may also be worthwhile. Immunohistochemical and histochemical analysis may also be used to identify specific cells or extracellular matrix and cellular activities in response to the bioactive materials.[65] Schoen discusses special considerations for the pathological evaluation of cardiovascular devices.[68]

Immobilization of an RGD-Containing Peptide: A Case Study

Described below is the sequence of testing that was done to determine the suitability of an arginine-glycine-aspartic acid (RGD)-containing peptide for the promotion of healing of cardiovascular medical textiles for applications such as sewing cuffs in mechanical heart valves. The materials modified were polyethylene terephthalate (PET) and polytetrafluoroethylene (PTFE) fabric. PET and PTFE textiles have shown good success when used in cardiovascular devices, however, the thrombogenic nature of PET and the nonadhesive nature of PTFE led to the exploration of what modification with an RGD-containing cell adhesion molecule would provide these textiles in terms of acceleration of a controlled healing.

Materials

Preparation of Substrates

PET films (Mylar®, DuPont) were cleaned using a series of ultrasonic baths in n-hexanes (J.T. Baker), ethanol (Pharmco), Sparkleen detergent (.1%, Fisher), and water (reverse osmosis (RO) purified) for 30 sec. each. PET fabrics (Meadox double velour, uncrimped, scoured and heatset; and Meadox® Woven Double Velour Dacron Graft) were used as received. PTFE fabric (Teflon®, Bard, U.S.C.) was used as received.

Peptide Source

The peptide investigated was PepTite™ Coating (PepTite, Telios Pharmaceuticals, Inc.). The amino acid sequence of PepTite is Ac-GRGDIPASSKGGGGSRLLLLLLR-NH_2 which consists of the cell binding domain, a spacer sequence and an adhesive poly leucine sequence. Its synthesis has been described.[22]

Coating and Sterilization of Substrates

PET and PTFE samples were coated in a dilute solution of the peptide (5-100 μg/ml, stock solution 5 mg/ml in DMSO) in phosphate buffered saline (Dulbeccos's, PBS) for a minimum of one hour with a low level of vacuum (25mmHg). Two, 30 min. rinses were done in PBS followed by two, 30 min. rinses in RO water. The coated substrates were then air dried in a laminar flow hood. Substrates were sterilized using steam for 40 min. at 121°C.

Cell Adhesion Assay

MG63 human osteosarcoma cells (ATCC) were used as a "quality control" cell line because of their expression of the appropriate integrins for the specific peptide studied. The cells were cultured in high glucose containing Dulbecco's modified eagle medium (DMEM, Gibco) with 10% fetal calf serum (Hyclone) 1% L-glutamine, and 100IU/ml penicillin/streptomycin (Gibco) at 37°C in 5% CO_2. Serum free medium consisted of DMEM containing 25 mM HEPES, and 1% ITS culture supplement (Collaborative Biomedical Products). Cells used in this assay were rinsed once with phophate buffered saline (PBS, 5ml for 75 cm^2 dish) and trypsinized. The trypsin was inhibited with 2.5 mg/ml soybean trypsin inhibitor (Gibco). Cells were centrifuged at 1000 rpm and resuspended in serum free medium. Samples were preblocked with serum free medium for a minimum of one hour. Cells (2×10^5) were added to each sample (approx. 1 cm^2) and incubated at 37°C for one hour in serum-free medium. After incubation, fabric was rinsed with PBS three times to remove loosely adherent cells. Attached cells were fixed in 3% formaldehyde, stained with 0.1% toluidine blue (TB) or crystal violet (CV) for 15 min. to overnight and rinsed with water. Controls were uncoated/unseeded and uncoated/seeded substrates. The number of cells attached were quantitated by solubilizing the stained cells using 1% sodium dodecylsulfate (SDS) and reading the absorbance of the dye at 630 nm (TB) or 595 nm (CV) wavelength as compared to the dye released from known numbers of stained cells.

Autoradiographic Assay

Radiolabelled PepTite (tritiated acetyl group) was used in autoradiographic assays to show coating uniformity and in coating stability assays. Autoradiograms were obtained by exposing substrates coated with tritiated peptide to film at -70°C for 24-72 hours.

ELISA (Enzyme-Linked Immunosorbent Assay)

This assay was used to monitor coating uniformity and density (qualitatively) without the need for radiolabels. Anti-PepTite™ antibodies were produced in rabbits using keyhole limpet hemocyanin (KLH) coupled to PepTite as the immunogen. PepTite free amines were coupled with sulfo-succinimidyl 4-N-maleimidomethyl cyclohexa NE-1-carboxylate (sulfo-SMCC, Pierce Chemical) yielding a maleamido functionality on the PepTite. A 20 fold excess of sulfo-SMCC was used in this reaction and unreacted material was separated from derivitized PepTite on a reverse phase HPLC column. Separately, KLH was thiolated by the use of 2-iminothiolane (Traut's reagent, Pierce Chemical) and excess thiolating reagent was removed by a desalting coumn (Sephadex G-25). The derivatized PepTite and thiolated KLH were allowed to react yielding a stable, covalent thioether bond. This material was used as the immunogen with no further purification.

Anti-PepTite™ antibody was purified using the Pierce™ ImmunoPure Plus Immobilized Protein A IgG Purification kit (no. 44679). ELISA assays were derived from Liddell and Cryer (1991) with the following exceptions. The wash buffer consisted of PBS containing 0.05% Tween 20 (Sigma), the blocking solution consisted of PBS containing 3% goat serum (Pierce), 1% ovalbumin (Sigma) and 1% casein (Pierce). The secondary antibody used was goat anti-rabbit IgG horseradish peroxidase conjugate (Pierce). The substrate that was used to form an insoluble colored end-product was DAB (3,3 diaminobenzidine tetrahydrochloride). The intensity of the color produced should correlate to the concentration of the primary antibody and the respective antigen.

Surface Analysis

The chemistry of modified PET film and fabric was analyzed using contact angle analysis and X-ray photoelectron spectroscopy (XPS). Contact angle analysis was performed on PET films with a Rame-Hart contact angle goniometer using the method of advancing contact angles. The critical surface tension (γ_c), dispersive and polar components of the surface free energy (γ_d and γ_p, respectively) were calculated by the methods of Zisman and Kaelble (1970 and 1964). XPS was performed on PET films and fabric using a Perkin Elmer Model 5500 XPS spectrometer. Average depth of penetration was 30 Å.

In Vitro Challenges

Stability Assay

Stability assays consisted of incubating tritiated peptide coated fabric in PBS or human plasma (whole blood was citrated 1:10 ratio and centrifuged at 2000 rpm) for 7-9 days at 37°C on a rocker table and determining the amount of coating remaining using a scintillation counter (Beckman).

Sterilization Challenge

This experiment consisted of subjecting coated PET and PTFE fabric to successive steam sterilization cycles to determine how many cycles the coating could withstand and still retain its activity. The coating activity and uniformity was assayed after the challenge using the cell adhesion assay and ELISA, respectively.

Arterial Patch

The arterial patch study was performed as described in Tweden et al (1995). Briefly four uncoated and coated PET and PTFE patches were implanted in the carotid and femoral arteries of dogs for 3 weeks. The animals were heparinized and their vessels containing the patches were perfusion fixed with 2% buffered glutaraldehyde, opened longitudinally, and portions for analysis were retrieved from the middle of the patch and along a longitudinal plane. Specimens were prepared for scanning electron microscopic and histological analysis using standard techniques. The thickness of neointima formed on the patches was quantitated with morphometric techniques.

Valve Replacement Model

Sewing cuffs were assembled using coated fabric under clean room conditions. The bioactivity was assessed using the cell adhesion assay and the uniformity was assessed using autoradiography (data not shown) after cuff assembly to ensure that an excessive amount of coating was not removed as a result of the assembly. St. Jude Medical® mechanical heart valves with either uncoated or PepTite coated polyester sewing cuffs were implanted in the mitral position in 16 juvenile sheep as described in Tweden et al.[79] No anticoagulants were given postoperatively. Between two to four weeks post implantation the valves were explanted after the animals were systemically anticoagulated with heparin. Explanted valves were fixed in Karnovsky's fixative and the sewing cuffs were analyzed grossly and histologically using semi-quantitative scales. Exposed Dacron, thrombus, thin pannus and pannus overgrowth were scored grossly from 0 to 5 in 15% or 25% intervals (0 poor response and 5 good response). Thin pannus is characterized by a smooth, white—appearing neointima under which the fabric pattern can still be seen. Pannus overgrowth is defined as tissue that begins to encroach on the valve orifice. Two samples for histological analysis were retrieved 180° apart (90° from the ear mechanism) and prepared using standard techniques. Histologic features graded were maturity and thickness of pannus (scale of 1-4 and in µm, respectively), presence of endothelial cells (+ or -), thrombus, deep organization, inflammation and calcification (scales of 0-4). The higher the score the poorer the response for the histological variables.

Results

In Vitro Assays

PepTite was found to consistently promote both cell attachment and spreading in serum-free medium to both PET and PTFE. In contrast, very few cells were found to attach to the uncoated samples and those that did had a round morphology (Figs. 8.1 and 8.2). Specifically, PepTite was shown to promote a 5 fold increase in cell attachment on the PET substrate as compared to its uncoated control and a 3.5 fold increase on the PTFE substrate as compared to its uncoated control (Fig. 8.3).

Both autoradiography and ELISA were used to assess the uniformity of the PepTite coating. Autoradiograms are shown in Figure 8.4. Close replications of the PET and PTFE fabric patterns were generated on the film indicating coating uniformity. Longer film exposures are needed for PTFE samples since it quenches radiation. Samples subjected to ELISA are also shown in Figure 8.4. The even brown color seen on PepTite coated PET samples indicates a relatively uniform coating. Results were similar on PTFE samples (data not shown).

The stability data for PepTite coated PET in plasma are shown in Figure 8.5. The coating was seen to be quite stable in both saline and plasma, with an initial minimal loss followed by a plateau. The amount of peptide remaining was found to promote cell attachment using the cell adhesion assay (data not shown). The amount of coating before the challenge was 157 µg/mg PET fabric and after 7 days of challenge was 119 µg/mg. The sterilization challenge showed that PepTite coated PET fabric could withstand five, 40 minute steam sterilization cycles (121°C, 15 psi) with no loss in coating uniformity or biological activity (evaluated with ELISA and cell adhesion assay, respectively, data not shown).

Contact angle analysis showed that PepTite modification of PET resulted in an increase in hydrophilicity, a decrease in critical surface tension (γ_c), and an increase in polarity (γ_p). Data are shown in Table 8.2. PepTite modified germanium was found to have similar surface energetics (Olivieri and Baier, 1994). The nitrogen (N)-containing amide bond of the peptide coating was shown by XPS. Also the higher the initial coating concentration, the higher the N signal seen by XPS (Table 8.3).

In Vivo Data

Scanning electron micrographs showing the typical healing response to the luminal side of uncoated and PepTite coated PET and PTFE patches are shown in Figures 8.6 and 8.7. On the uncoated patches, the response is characterized by a platelet/fibrin matt, rounded leukocytes and spreading cells which appear to be macrophages. In contrast, the PepTite coated patches were characterized by a complete lining of the luminal side by cells that had surface

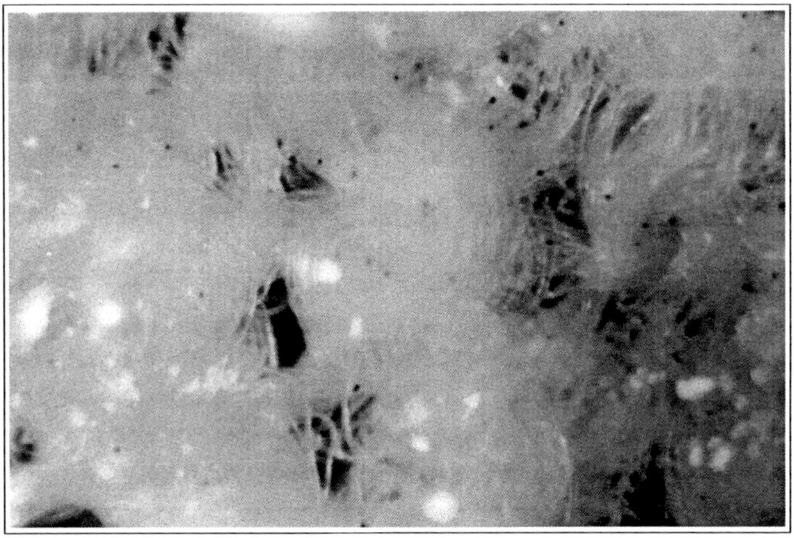

Fig. 8.1A. Cell attachment to uncoated PET fabric.

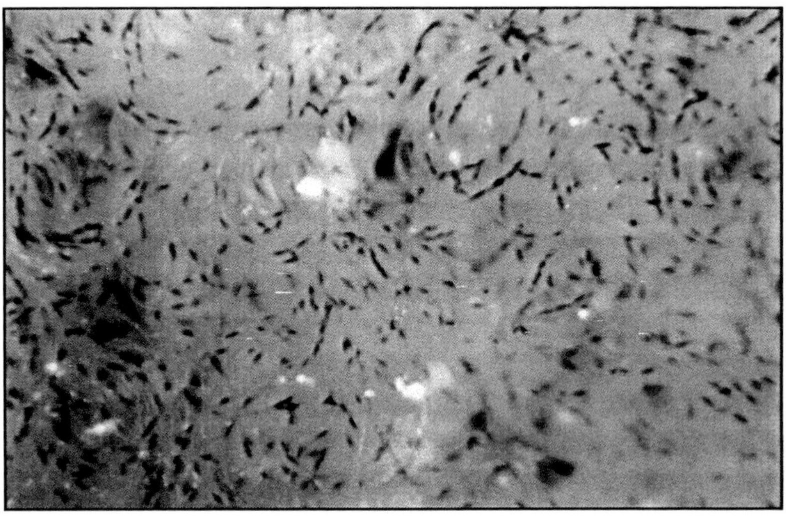

Fig. 8.1B. Cell attachment to PepTite coated PET fabric using cell adhesion assay described above.

morphology characteristic of endothelial cells (Figs. 8.6B and 8.7B). The morphological characterization showed that 75% (3 out of 4) of the PepTite coated patches were covered with endothelial-like cells whereas only 25% (1 out of 4) of the uncoated patches had a similar lining. Openings of vasa vasorum which are lined with elongated endothelial-like cells were seen on the healed surfaces.

Typical histological sections through the explanted patches are seen in Figure 8.8. These sections were taken longitudinally, so that the characteristic hills and valleys of the crimped fabric pattern can be seen. The measurements for the neointimal thickness were taken along the patch at the "hills" of the graft away from the anastomosis. The neointimal thickness

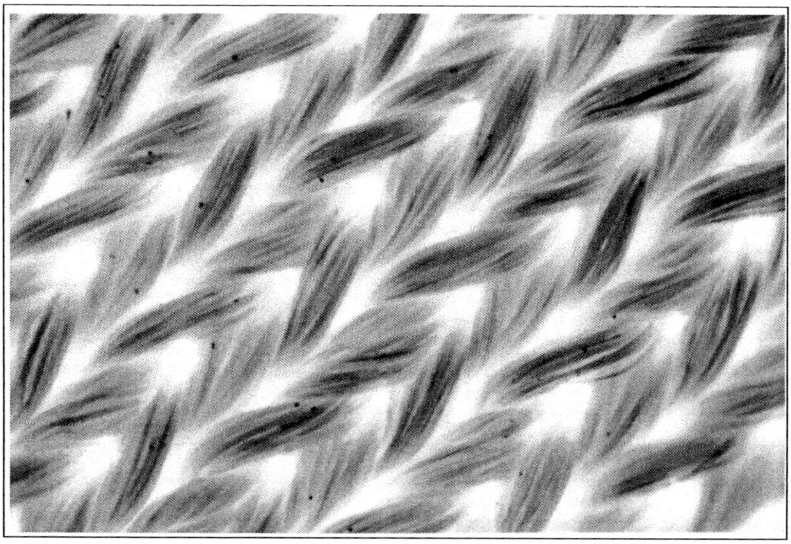

Fig. 8.2A. Cell attachment to uncoated PTFE fabric

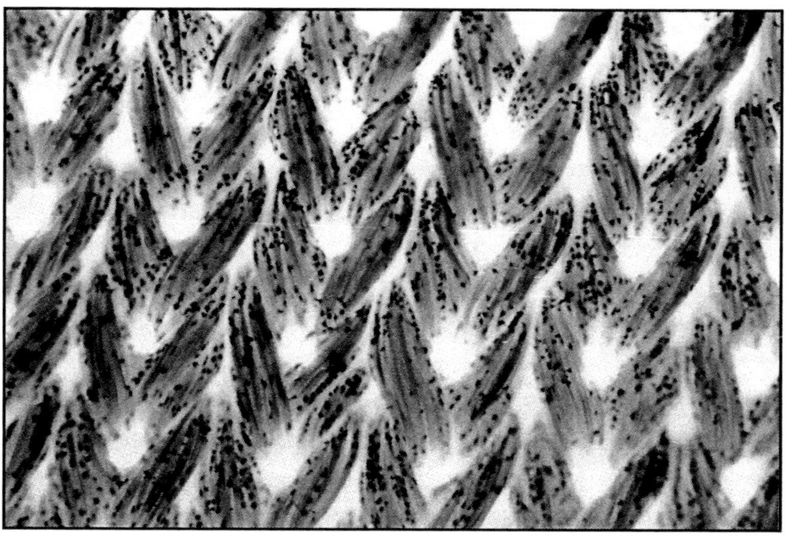

Fig. 8.2B. Cell attachment to PepTite coated PTFE fabric using cell adhesion assay described above.

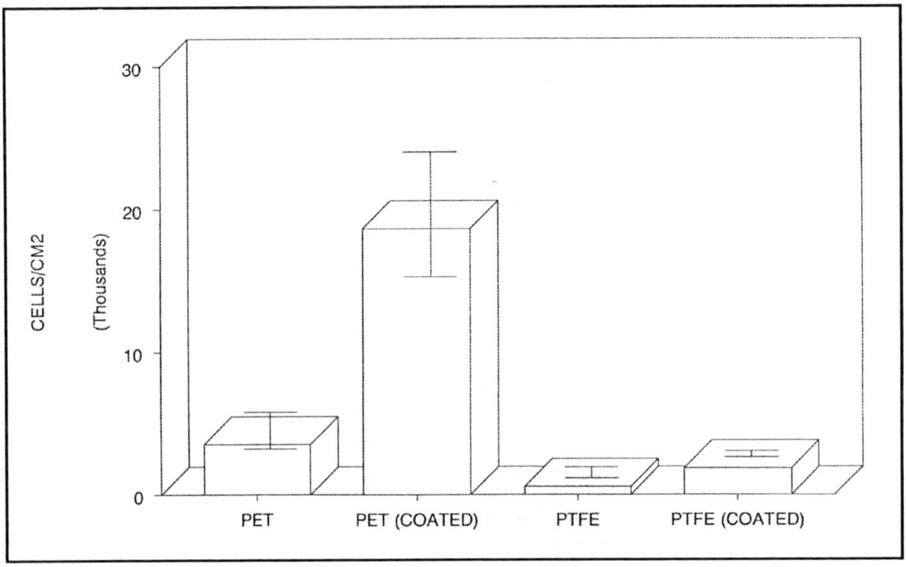

Fig. 8.3. Graph showing quantitation of cell attachment using a colorimetric method.

Fig. 8.4. Top two rows: Autoradiogram of PepTite coated PET fabric (left) and PTFE fabric (right, top row is 24 hr exposure to film, second row is 1 week exposure to film), bottom row: ELISA of uncoated (left two) and coated PET fabric (right two).

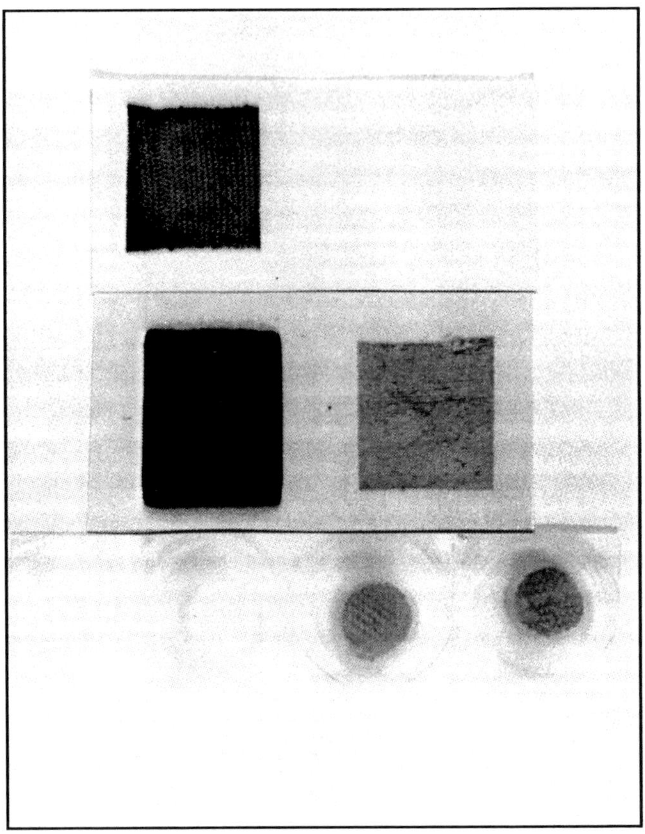

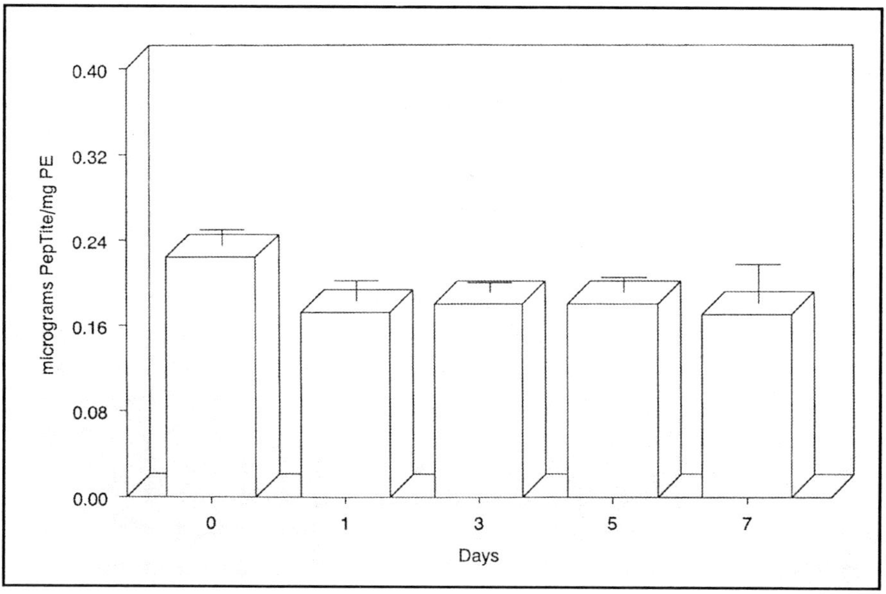

Fig. 8.5. Coating stability in plasma

Table 8.2. Contact angle analysis of PepTite modified Mylar® PET

Sample (n)	Conc. PepTite (μg/ml)	Y_c (dynes/cm) (SD)	Y_p (dynes/cm) (SD)	Y_d (dynes/ cm) (SD)	Water Contact Angle(°)(SD)
PET (n = 3)	0	40.0	6.9	31.6	85
		(3.4)	(1.2)	(3.0)	(10)
PET (n = 2)	5	35.5	19.1	23.6	62
		(3.8)	(0.4)	(1.0)	(0)
PET (n = 2)	50	33.9	16.1	26.3	62
		(0.5)	(0.8)	(1.0)	(0)

measurements showed that the pannus thickness on PepTite coated PET patches was essentially half of that seen on uncoated patches (mean of 120 vs 66 μm). No difference in neointimal thickness was seen between uncoated and PepTite coated PTFE patches. The extent of foreign body giant cells seen associated with the PET fibers was reduced noticeably in the PepTite coated PET patches as compared to the uncoated patches (Figs. 8.8A and 8.8B).

Representative gross macrographs of valves with uncoated and PepTite coated polyester cuffs explanted at approximately 2.4 weeks are shown in Figure 8.9. The uncoated cuff healing was characterized by thrombus build-up and exposed Dacron fabric. In contrast, the coated cuff healing was characterized by a greater amount of white, smooth pannus that appeared endothelialized at this time period. Overall, the significant differences seen in the gross and histological data were the following: a greater extent of thin pannus formation on the inflow side of the coated cuffs compared to that on the uncoated cuffs (mean of 4.1 and 2.1, respectively, $p < 0.001$), a 27% thicker pannus on the uncoated cuffs (411 mm) compared to that

Table 8.3. Atomic concentrations (%) of PepTite modified Dacron® and Mylar® (standard deviation)

Sample	C	O	Si	N	F	Na	Cl
Dacron (n = 3)	72.7 (1.3)	27.1 (1.2)	0.16 (0.09)	–	–	ND	ND
Dacron 5 μg/ml PepTite (n = 2)	70.8 (0.85)	25.9 (0.9)	0.2 (0)	3.2 (0.1)	0.1*	–	–
Mylar (n = 2)	87.3 (14.9)	12.3 (14.5)	0.5 (0.3)	–	–	ND	ND
Mylar 5 μg/ml PepTite (n = 2)	72.7 (2.4)	23.4 (2.7)	1.0 (0.4)	3.0 (0.6)	–	–	–
Mylar 50 μg/ml PepTite (n = 3)	74.3 (7.3)	21.3 (6.9)	0.5 (0.1)	4.0 (0.4)	–	–	–

* = detected in one sample only.
ND = not determined.

seen on the coated cuffs (301 mm, p=0.04), and finally, more advanced pannus maturity on the coated cuffs at 3 weeks (1.9) than that seen on the uncoated cuffs (2.6, p=0.04). These findings indicated an accelerated and more controlled healing to the PepTite coated PET sewing cuffs compared to that seen with the uncoated cuffs (Table 8.4).

Discussion

The methods for the testing of materials modified with bioactive molecules for medical devices were outlined. Results using the outlined testing strategy on fabrics modified with an RGD-containing peptide for use in cardiovascular devices were discussed. First it was shown that the coated fabric had acceptable bioactivity using the cell line MG63 osteosarcoma. PepTite has also been shown to promote the attachment and spreading of an endothelial cell line which is a cell type more relevant to the tissue of interest (data not shown). The coating was shown to be uniform in nature using the autoradiogram assay and ELISA which was shown to be important for uniform cell response (data not shown). The coating amount was quantitated using radiolabelled peptide. This technique could also be used to determine the minimum amount of coating needed for adequate biological activity. The chemical nature and surface energetics of the coating were analyzed using XPS (the coating could be seen with the presence of a N peak) and contact angle analysis (the coating was more hydrophilic and polar in nature than the substrate), respectively. It was found that the coating could not be detected using either scanning electron microscopic or ATR-IR analysis since only low concentrations were needed for acceptable biological activity on the materials (data not shown). The coating was also shown to be able to withstand biologic (buffer and plasma shaker bath storage) and manufacturing (successive sterilization cycles and fabrication into cuff prototypes) challenges with little decrease in coating activity. Finally, the "ultimate" challenge of in vivo biological activity using a simple vascular patch model and a valve replacement model showed that the coating accelerated wound healing corroborating the in vitro cell adhesion data. The biological significance of such a coating in a mechanical heart valve application is discussed elsewhere.[79]

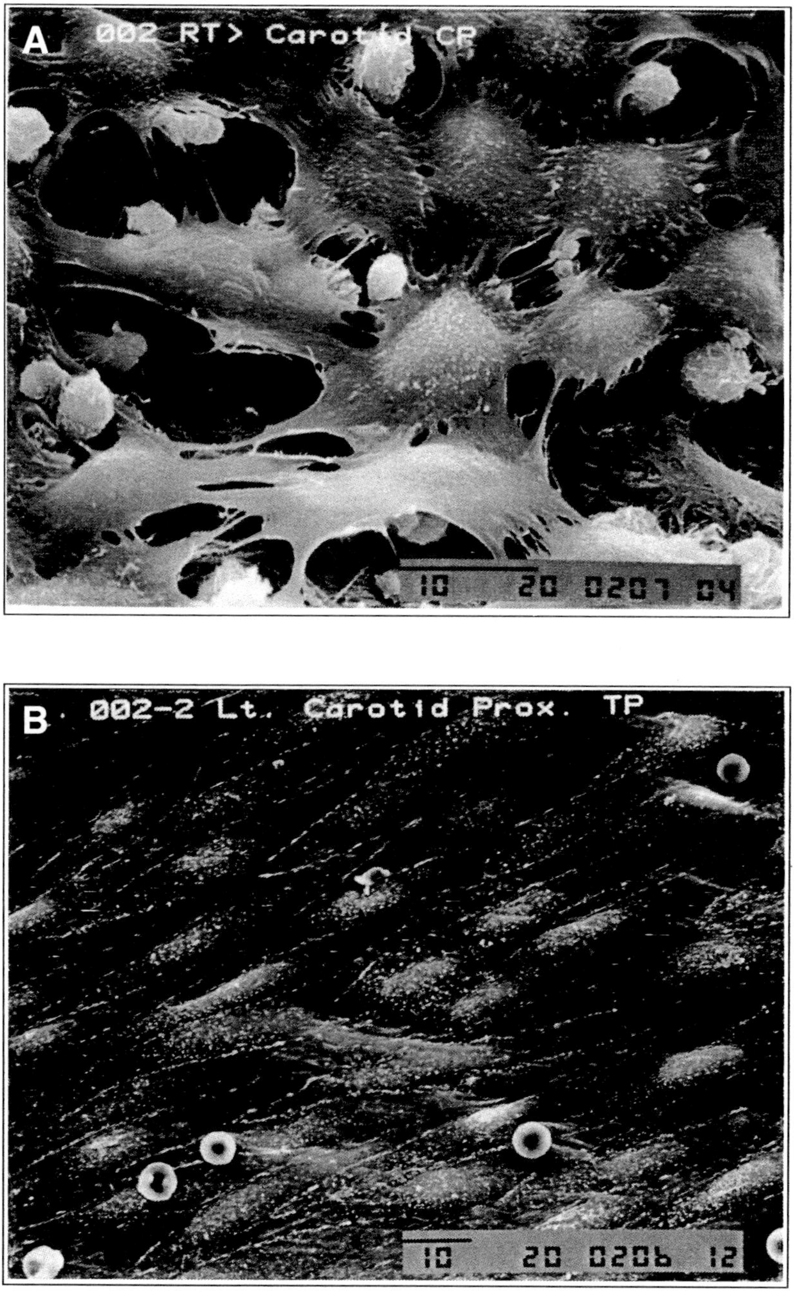

Figs. 8.6A,B. Scanning electron micrograph of luminal side of explanted A) uncoated PET and B) coated PET vascular patch.

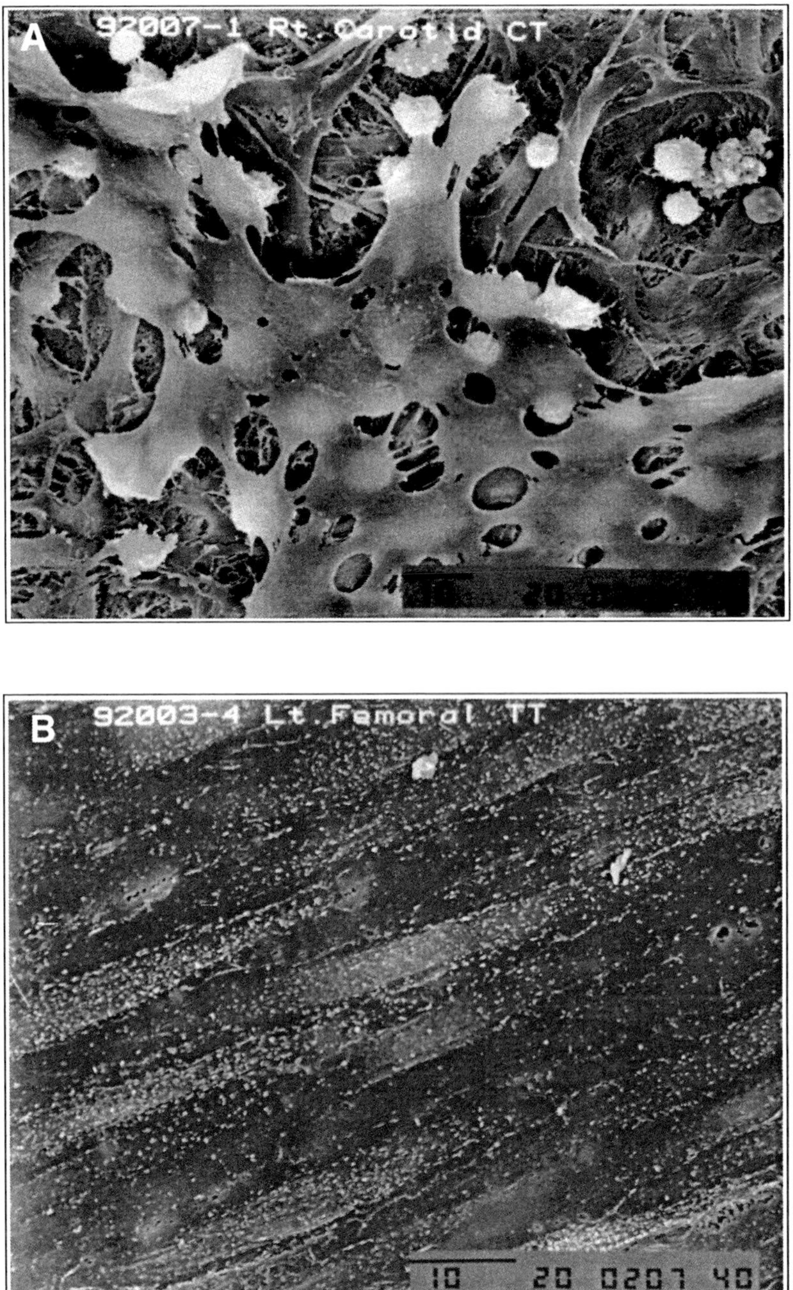

Fig. 8.7. Scanning electron micrograph of luminal side of explanted A) uncoated PTFE and B) coated PTFE vascular patch.

Table 8.4. Valve replacement model significant gross and histological data

Sample	Gross Thin Pannus	Histologic Pannus Thick (μm)	Histologic Pannus Maturity
Uncoated	2.1[a]	411[b]	2.6[c]
PepTite coated	4.1	301	1.9

a $p < 0.001$, b $p = 0.04$, c $p = 0.04$

In conclusion, a full range of testing is necessary to determine on a case-by-case basis if materials modified with bioactive molecules can be used successfully in medical devices.

Acknowledgements

Thanks are extended to Sheila Kelly and Dan Langanki (St. Jude Medical) for performing cell adhesion assays, ELISA, and sterilization challenges. Thanks are also extended to former and present personnel from Telios that performed radioisotope studies and were involved in the in vitro work direction, specifically Jonathan Blevitt, James Glass, Kenneth Dickerson, William Craig, Ph.D., and Michael Pierschbacher, Ph.D.. Hiroaki Harasaki, M.D., Ph.D. from the Cleveland Clinic Foundation performed the vascular patch study and Michael Jones, M.D. from the NIH performed the valve study.

References

1. Axelrod D, Thompson NL, Burghart TP. Total internal reflection fluorescence microscopy. J Microscopy 1982; 129:19-28.
2. Bernex F, Mazzucotelli JP, Roudiere JL et al. In vitro endothelialization of carbon-coated dacron vascular grafts. Intl J Artif Organs 1992; 15:172-180.
3. Black J. Biological Performance of Materials. New York: Marcel Dekker, Inc. 1992: 301-329.
4. Blawas AS, Reichert WM. Patterning antibodies on surfaces for a multiple analyte sensor. Surfaces in Biomaterials Symposium 1995: 39-43.
5. Block SS. Disinfection, Sterilization, and Preservation. 4th edition. Philadelphia:Lea & Febiger, 1991.
6. Burgess WH, Maciag T. The heparin-binding (fibroblast) gorwth factor family of proteins. Annu Rev Biochem 1989; 58:575-606.
7. Burridge K, Fath K, Kelly T et al. Focal adhesions: Transmembrane junctions between the extracellular matrix and the cytoskeleton. A Rev Cell Biol 1988; 4:487-525.
8. Cameron BL, Tsuchida H, Connall TP et al. High porosity PTFE improves endothelialization of arterial grafts without increasing early thrombogenicity. J Cardiovasc Surg 1993; 34:282-285.
9. Cappello J, Crissman J, Dorman M et al. Genetic engineering of structural protein polymers. Biotechnol Prog 1990; 6:198-202.
10. Cholvin NR. General compatibility assessment. In: Von Recum, AF ed. Handbook of Biomaterials Evaluation. New York: Macmillan Publishing Co. 1986: 293-305.
11. Cook SD, Thomas KA, Brinker MR. Bioactive ceramic coatings for orthopaedic and dental implant applications. In: Sharma CP, Szycher M, eds. Blood Compatible Materials and Devices. Lancaster, Pennsylvania: Technomic Publish Co., Inc. 1991:279-287.

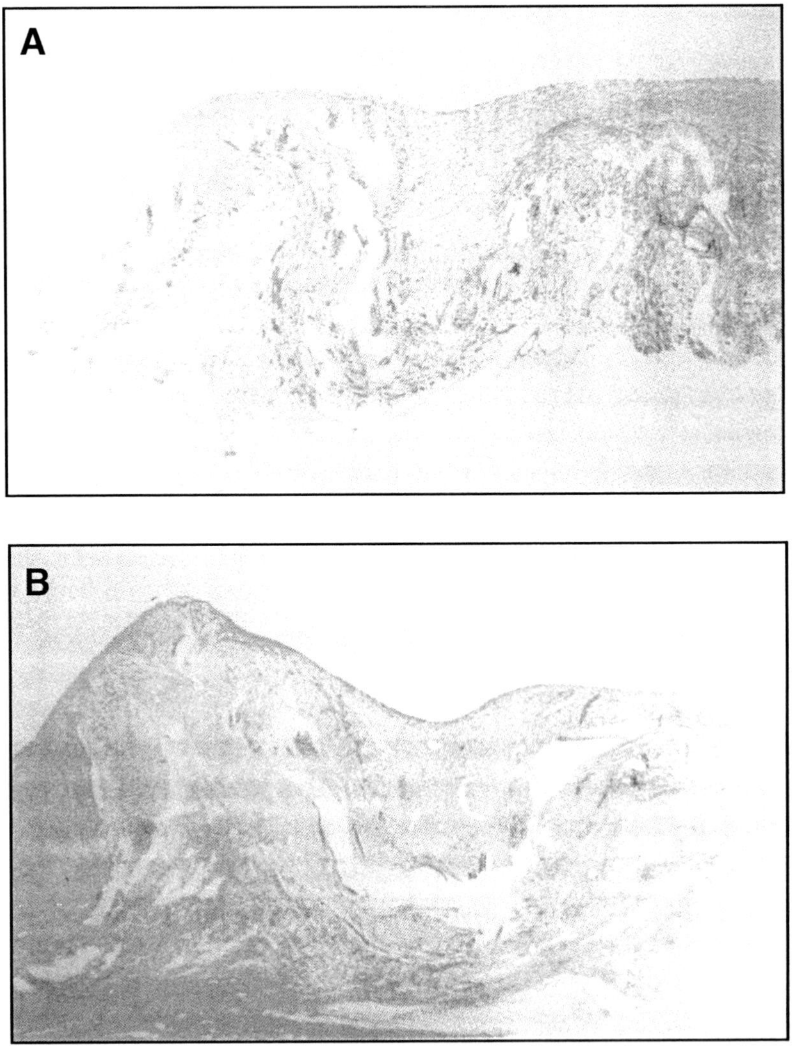

Figs. 8.8. A) Histological section of uncoated PET vascular patch, B) Histological section of coated PET vascular patch.

12. Danilich MJ, Gervasio D, Marchant RE. Preparation and characterization of active glucose oxidase immobilized to a plasma-polymerized film. In: Edelman PG, Wang J, eds. Biosensors and Chemical Sensors, ACS Series 1992; 487:84-98.
13. Desai NP, Hubbell JA. Surface physical interpenetrating networds of poly(ethylene terephthalate) and poly(ethylene oxide) with biomedical applications. Macromolecules 1992; 25:226-232.
14. Doillon CJ, Côté M-F, Pietrucha K et al. Porosity and biological properties of polyethylene glycol-conjugated collagen materials. J Biomater Sci Polymer Edn 1994; 6:715-728.
15. Dunkirk SG, Gregg SL, Duran LW et al. Photochemical coatings for the prevention of bacterial colonization. J Biomater Appl 1991; 6:131-156.
16. Ebert CD, Kim SW. Immobilized heparin: Spacer arm effects on biological interactions. Thrombosis Res 1982; 26:43-57.

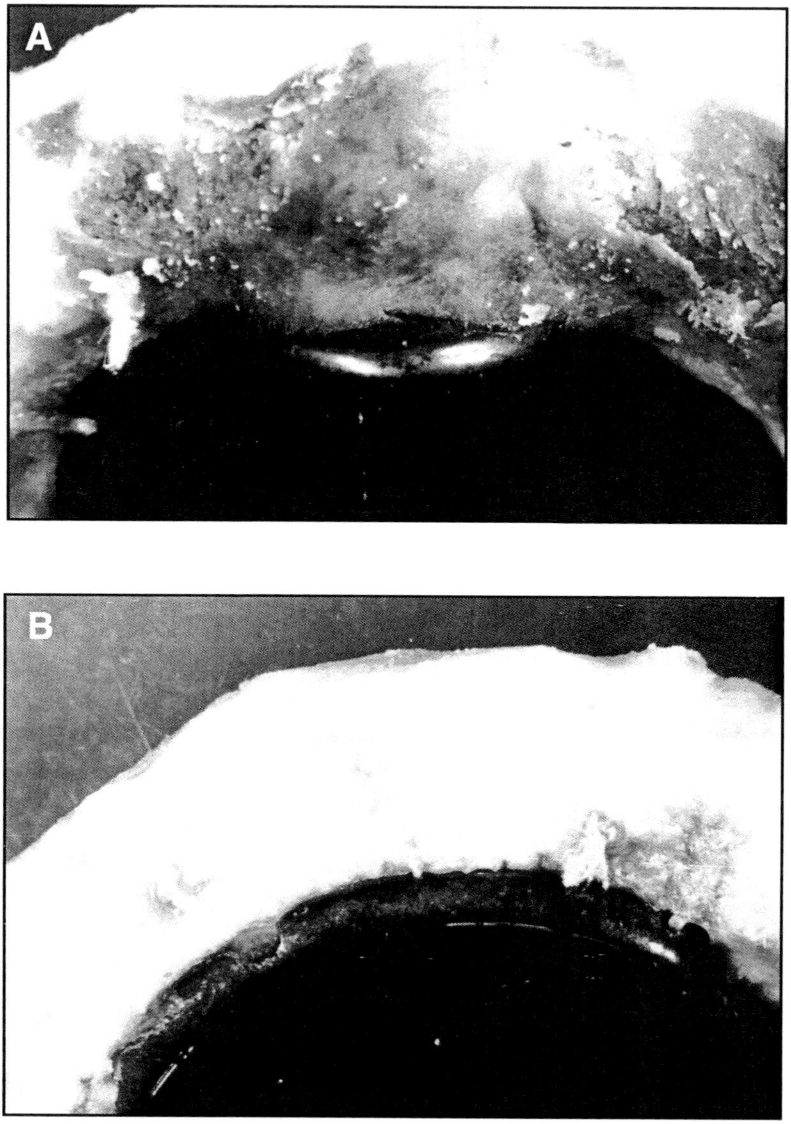

Figs. 8.9. A) Mechanical heart valve explant with uncoated PET sewing cuff, B) Mechanical heart valve explant with coated PET sewing cuff.

17. Edmunds LH. Thrombotic and bleeding complications of prosthetic heart valves. Ann Thorac Surg 1987; 44:430-445.
18. Eppell SJ, Simmons SR, Albrecht RM et al. Cell-surface receptors and proteins on platelet membranes imaged by scanning force microscopy using immunogold contrast enhancement. Biophysical J 1995; 68:671-680.
19. Fischlein T, Fasol R. In vitro endothelialization of bioprosthetic heart valves. J Heart Valve Dis 1996; 5:58-65.

20. Garfinkle AM, Hoffman AS, Ratner BD et al. Effects of a tetrafluoroethylene glow discharge on patency of small diameter dacron vascular grafts. Trans Am Soc Artif Organs 1984; 30:432-439.
21. Gingell D, Todd I. Interference reflection microscopy. A quantitative theory for image interpretation and its application to cell-substratum separation measurements. Biophs J 1979; 26:507-526.
22. Glass J, Blevitt J, Dickerson K et al. Cell attachment and mobility on materials modified by surface active RGD containing peptides. Ann NY Acad Sci 1994; 523:177-186.
23. Goodman SL, Tweden KS, Albrecht RM. Three-dimensional morphology and platelet adhesion on pyrolytic carbon heart valve materials. Cells and Materials 1995; 5:15-30.
24. Goodman SL, Park K, Albrecht RM. A correlative approach to colloidal gold labeling with video-enhanced light microscopy, low-voltage scanning electron microscopy, and high-voltage electron microscopy. Colloidal Gold: Principles, Methods, and Applications 1991; 3:369-409.
25. Gosselin C, Vorp DA, Warty V et al. ePTFE coating with fibrin glue, FGF-1, and heparin: effect on retention of seeded endothelial cells. J Surg Res 1996; 60:327-332.
26. Gosselin C, Ren D, Ellinger J et al. In vivo platelet deposition on polytetrafluorethylene coated with fibrin glue containing fibroblast growth factor 1 and heparin in a canine model. Am J Surg 1995; 170:126-130.
27. Greisler HP, Klosak JJ, Dennis JW et al. Biomaterial pretreatment with ECGF to augment endothelial cell proliferation. J Vasc Surg 1987; 5:393-399.
28. Harrick NJ. Internal Reflection Spectroscopy. Harrick Scientific Corp., Ossing, New York, 1979.
29. Harlow E, Lane D. Antibodies: A Laboratory Manual. New York:Cold Spring Harbor Laboratory, 1988.
30. Haugland RP. Handbook of fluorescent probes and research chemicals. Larison KD (ed.) Molecular Probes, Inc. Eugene OR, 5th edition 1992.
31. Hercules DM. Surface analysis of organic material with TOF-SIMS. J Mol Structure 1993; 292:49-64.
32. Hirsch D, Drader J, Pathak YV et al. Synergistic inhibition of the calcification of glutaraldehyde pretreated bovine pericardium in a rat subdermal model by $FeCl_3$ amd ethanehydroxydiphosphonate: preincubation and polymeric controlled release studies. Biomaterials 1993; 14:705-710.
33. Hoffman A. Modification of material surfaces to affect how they interact with blood. In: Leonard EF, Turitto VT, Vroman L, eds. Blood in Contact with Natural and Artificial Surfaces. Ann NY Acad Sci 1987; 516:96-101.
34. Horbett TA, Waldburger JJ, Ratner BD, Hoffman AS. Cell adhesion to a series of hydrophilic-hydrophobic copolymers studied with a spinning disc apparatus. J Biomed Mater Res 1988; 22:383-404.
35. Hubbell JA. Pharmacologic modification of materials. Cardiovasc Pathol 1993; 2:121S-127S.
36. Hubbell JA Massia SP, Desai NP et al. Endothelial cell-selective materials for tissue engineering in the vascular graft via a new receptor. Bio/Technology 1991; 9:586-572.
37. Huebsch JB, Fields GB, Triebes TG et al. Photoreactive analog of peptide FN-C/H-V from the carboxy-terminal heparin-binding domains of fibronectin supports endothelial cell adhesion and spreading on biomaterial surfaces. J Biomed Mater Res 1996; 31:555-567.
38. Huebsch JC, McCarthy JB, Diglio CA et al. Endothelial cell interactions with synthetic peptides from the carboxy-terminal heparin-binding domains of fibronectin. Circ Res 1995; 77:43-53.
39. Ito Y, Liu L-S, Matsuo R et al. Synthesis and nonthrombogenicity of polymer membrane with surface-graft polymers carrying thrombin inhibitor. J Biomed Mater Res 1992a; 26:1065-1080.
40. Ito Y, Liu S-Q, Nakabayashi M et al. Cell growth on immobilized cell-growth factor. Biomaterials 1992b; 13:789-794.
41. Jacobs HA, Okano T, Kim SW. Antithrombogenic surfaces: characterization and bioactivity of surface immobilized PGE_1-heparin conjugate. J Biomed Mater Res 1989; 23:611-630.
42. Jansen B, Rinck M, Wolbring P et al. In vitro evaluation of the antimicrobial efficacy and biocompatibility of a silver-coated central venous catheter. J Biomater App 1994; 9:55-70.
43. Kaelble DH. Dispersion-polar surface tension properties of organic solids. J Adhesion 1970; 2:66-81.
44. Kemeny DM. A practical guide to ELISA. New York: Pergamon Press, 1991.
45. Kottke-Marchant K, Anderson JM, Umemura Y et al. Effect of albumin coating on the in vitro blood compatibility of Dacron arterial prostheses. Biomaterials 1989; 10:147-155.

46. Leonard EF, Turitto VT, Vroman L, eds. Blood in Contact with Natural and Artificial Surfaces. Annals New York Acad Sci 1987; 517:1-688.
47. Lewinsohn DM, Nickologg BJ, Butcher EC. A fluorometric approach to the quantitation of cell number with application to a cell adhesion assay. J Immunological research 1988; 110:93-100.
48. Levy RJ, Schoen FJ, Anderson HC et al. Cardiovascular implant calcification: a survey and update. Biomaterials 1991; 12:707-714.
49. Liddell JE, Cryer A. A Practical Guide to Monoclonal Antibodies. England: John Wiley and Sons ltd., 1991.
50. Lowenberg BF, Pilliar RM, Aubin JE et al. Cell attachment of human gingival fibroblasts in vitro to porous-surfaced titanium alloy discs coated with collagen and platelet-derived growth factor. Biomaterials 1988; 9:302-309.
51. Machin D, Campbell MJ. Statistical Tables for the Design of Clinical Trials. Boston: Blackwell Scientific Publications, 1987.
52. Marchant RE, Lea AS, Andrade JD et al. Interactions of von willebrand factor on mica studied by atomic force microscopy. J Colloid and Interface Sci 1992; 148:261-272.
53. Miki M, dos Remedios CG. Fluorescence quenching studies of fluorescein attached to Lys-61 or Cys-374 in actin: Effects of polymerization, myosin subfragment-1 binding and tropomyosin-troponin binding. J Biochem 1988; 104:232-235.
54. Natiella JR. Odontocompatibility assessment. In: Von Recum A, ed. Handbook of Biomaterials Evaluation. New York: Macmillan Publishing Co., 1986:339-348.
55. Nilles JL, Karagianes MT, Wheeler KR. Porous titanium alloy for fixation of knee prostheses. J Biomed Mater Res Symp 1974; 5:319-328.
56. Northrup SJ. Mammalian Cell Culture. In: Von Recum A, ed. Handbook of Biomaterials Evaluation. New York: Macmillan Publishing Co., 1986:209-225.
57. O'Neal RB, Sauk JJ, Somerman MJ. Biological requirements for material integration. J Oral Implantology 1992; 18:243-255.
58. Ozaki CK, Phaneuf MD, Bide MJ et al. In vivo testing of an infection-resistant vascular graft material. J Surg Res 1993; 55:543-547.
59. Olivieri MP, Rittle KH, Tweden KS et al. Comparative biophysical study of adsorbed calf serum, fetal bovine serum and mussel adhesive protein films. Biomaterials 1992; 13:201-208.
60. Olivieri MP, Baier RE. Conformation of a cell attachment peptide to a model surface. Society for Biomaterials 20th meeting abstracts 1994:344.
61. Patel BCM, Courtney JM, Evans JH et al. Biocompatibility assessment: Application of fluorescent probe response (FPR) techniques. Biomaterials 1991; 12:722-726.
62. Ragnarson B, Bengtsson L, Hægerstrand A. Labeling with fluorescent carbocyanine dyes of cultured endothelial and smooth muscle cells by growth in dye-containing medium. Histochemistry 1992; 97:329-333.
63. Ratner BD. Surface characterization of materials for blood contact applications. In: Cooper SL, Peppas NA, eds. Biomaterials: Interfacial Phenomena and Applications. ACS 1982;199:9-24.
64. Ripamonti U, Ma SS, van den Heever B et al. Osteogenin, a bone morphogenetic protein, adsorbed on porous hydroxyapatite substrata, induces rapid bone differentiation in calvarial defects in adult primates. Plast Reconstr Surg 1992; 90:3820393.
65. Salthouse TN. Histochemical and quantitative microscopy. In: Von Recum A, ed. Handbook of Biomaterials Evaluation. New York: Macmillan Publishing Co., 1986:398-407.
66. Salzman EW, Merrill EW. Interaction of blood with artificial surfaces. In: Colman RW, Hirsh J, Marder VJ, Salzman EW, eds. Hemostasis and Thrombosis. 2nd ed. Philadelphia: J.B. Lippincott Co., 1987:1335-1347.
67. Sawyer PN, Sophie Z, O'Shaughnessy AM. Hemocompatibility assessment. In: Von Recum A, ed. Handbook of Biomaterials Evaluation. New York: Macmillan Publishing Co. 1986: 306-320.
68. Schoen FJ. Special considerations for pathological evaluation of explanted cardiovascular prostheses. In: Von Recum A, ed. Handbook of Biomaterials Evaluation. New York: Macmillan Publishing Co. 1986:412-435.
69. Schwartz ML, Sheldon D, Dorman F et al. Local anticoagulation of prosthetic heart valves. Circulation 1973; XLVIII, Supplement III:111-85-89.

70. Sefton MV, Cholakis CH, Llanos G. Preparation of nonthrombogenic materials by chemical modification. In: Williams DF, ed. Blood Compatibility. Boca Raton: CRC Press, Inc., 1987; 1:151-198.
71. Sheehan C. Clinical Immunology. Philadelphia: J.B. Lippincott Co., 1990.
72. Sioshansi P. New processes for surface treatment of catheters. Artif Organs 1994; 18:266-271.
73. Smith PK, Mallia AK, Hermanson GT. Colorimetric method for the assay of heparin content in immobilized heparin preparations. Analytical Biochem 1980; 109:466-473.
74. Swier P, Bos WJ, Mohammad SF et al. An in vitro test model to study the performance and thrombogenecity of cardiovascular devices. ASAIO Trans 1989; 35:683-687.
75. Talbot MD, Ambler J, Butler KD et al. Recombinant desulphatohirudin (CGP 39393) anticoagulant and antithrombotic properties in vivo. Thrombosis and Hemostasis 1989; 61:77-80.
76. Tencer AF, Holmes RE, Johnson KD. Osteocompatibility assessment. In: Von Recum A, ed. Handbook of Biomaterials Evaluation. New York: Macmillan Publishing Co., 1986:321-338.
77. Turitto VT, Leonard EF. Platelet adhesion to a spinning surface. Trans Amer Soc Artif Int Organs 1972; XVIII:348-354.
78. Tweden KS, Spadone DP, Terranova VP. Neovascularization on surface demineralized dentin. J Periodont 1989; 60:460-466.
79. Tweden KS, Harasaki H, Jones M et al. Accelerated Healing of Cardiovascular Textiles promoted by a RGD peptide. J Heart Valve Disease 1995; 4 (Suppl. I):S90-S97.
80. Vulic I, Okano T, Kim SW. Synthesis and characterization of polystyrene-poly(ethylene oxide)-heparin block copolymers. J Poly Sci Part A: Polymer Chem 1988; 26:381-391.
81. Walenga JM, Hoppensteadt D, Fareed J et al. Hemostatic abnormalities in total artificial heart patients as detected by specific blood markers. Ann Thorac Surg 1992; 53:844-850.
82. Yamamura K, Sakurai T, Yano K et al. Sustained release of basic fibroblast growth factor from the synthetic vascular prosthesis using hydroxypropylchitosan acetate. J Biomed Mater Res 1995; 19:203-206.
83. Yuan S, Cai W, Szakalas-Gratzl G et al. Immobilization of heparin oligosaccharides onto radiofrequency plasma modified pyrolytic carbon-coated graphite. J App Biomat 1995; 6:259-266.
84. Zidovetzki R, Yarden Y, Schlessinger J et al. Rotational diffusion of epidermal growth factor complexed to cell surface receptors reflects rapid microaggregation anad endocytosis of occupied receptors. Proc Natl Acad Sci 1981; 78:6981-6985.
85. Zisman WA. Relation of the equilibrium contact angle to liquid and constitution. Adv Chem Ser 1964; 43:1-51.

APPENDIX

Selecting Contract Labs

Barry Sall

1. FDA compliance history: The lab should give prospective clients copies of documentation from recent FDA inspections. If not, these are available through FDA FOI, but it takes time. There are quicker sources for warning letters.
2. Visit the lab: If the lab houses animals, the first impression one obtains is smell. Also check facilities, documentation systems, sample archives and the QAU. Meet with people that actually perform the work and determine their level of technical ability.
3. References: Can you speak with other firms that have used the lab's services? Discussions with colleauges at professional meetings can also be good sources of information on contract lab capabilities.
4. The bidding process I: Draw up a brief specification sheet describing each test, the number of samples or animals used, follow up or observation times, analytical techniques employed and reporting requirements. This increases the likelihood that when comparing competitive bids, you will compare "apples with apples".
5. The bidding process II: The lowest bidder is not always the least expensive lab. "Doing it right the first time" is vital. Experienced labs require less direction and can often provide useful advice to research sponsors.
6. Auditing: Will the contract lab permit auditing during the study? This is a good way to confirm progress and data quality, especially for long term studies.

Biomaterials in the Design and Reliability of Medical Devices, edited by Michael N. Helmus

Index

A

Antioxidant 118, 123, 125, 150
ASTM 2, 3, 5-51, 53, 56-67, 107, 118, 149

B

Bioactive molecules 201, 202, 207, 217, 220
Bioavailability 108, 111, 125
Biocompatibility 2-5, 20, 24, 30, 46, 53, 54, 56, 63, 68, 69, 74, 105-107, 113-115, 118, 124, 125, 147, 149-153, 155, 158, 173, 184, 185, 187, 189
Bioprosthetic 13, 27, 28, 32, 42, 59, 202

C

Calibration 144, 145, 191, 192
Carcinogenicity 5, 56, 107, 113-115, 121, 124, 125, 147, 149, 158, 160, 165-168, 173
Catheters 2, 4, 13-16, 19-22, 25, 53, 55, 57, 58, 62, 67, 124, 128, 155, 158, 186, 201
CEN 3, 8, 132
Ceramics 1, 66, 70, 72, 107, 168, 169, 180
Characterization 2, 14-16, 19, 33, 55, 74, 107, 108, 111, 112, 114, 118, 124, 125, 150-153, 169, 175, 181, 184, 202, 203, 213
Chemicals of concern 112
Chitosan 61, 73, 167
Contact angle analysis 204, 205, 211, 212, 217
Cyclohexanone 119
Cytotoxicity 2, 4, 5, 28, 68, 107, 118, 125, 141, 142, 148-150, 152, 153, 155, 157, 173, 206

D

Degradation 4-6, 10, 42, 45, 49, 55-61, 68, 111, 113, 115, 123-125, 150, 163, 168-170, 175, 178, 179
Design controls 130, 173
Design history 130, 131, 182, 183, 192
Design review 131
Device classification 125
Devices 1-51, 53, 54, 56-59, 63, 69, 75, 127, 147, 187, 190-192, 194, 195, 197, 201, 202, 206-209, 217, 220
Durability 1, 3, 4, 46, 55, 57, 62, 63, 74, 130, 172, 175, 178-180

E

Explants 175, 209
Extraction 5, 6, 108, 111-113, 118, 123, 124, 148-152, 169, 173, 185

F

Facilities 143, 172, 182, 184
Fatigue 1, 3, 11, 17, 38, 40, 42, 46, 50, 55, 57, 58, 59, 63, 66, 67, 175, 178-180, 189
FDA 2, 3, 5-54, 57, 69-74, 105-108, 118, 124, 127, 128, 130-133, 141-145, 150, 158, 170-172, 180-183, 185, 186, 188-190, 193-196
Functional requirements 3, 55

G

Genotoxicity 5, 106, 113, 115, 121, 125, 141, 147, 149, 150, 160, 163, 165, 167, 168, 173
Guidance documents 2, 54, 105, 107, 130, 131, 133, 142, 170, 173, 195
Guidelines 2-51, 53, 56, 57, 74, 106, 125, 158, 165, 167, 168, 170, 173, 180

H

Hemocompatibility 125, 141, 149, 159, 162, 163, 165-167, 172, 173, 209
Hemodialyzer 19, 107, 151, 158, 172
Hydrogels 25, 27, 28, 57, 62, 71
Hydrolysis 55, 124, 169
Hyperplasia 2, 11, 22, 121, 122, 166, 178, 201

I

IDE 14, 15, 17, 27, 42, 105, 127, 128, 131, 183, 190
Immunotoxicity 9, 113, 132, 149, 153, 154, 155, 157
Implant tissue interface 125, 165, 178
Implants 1, 2, 6, 8, 11, 13, 19, 20, 22, 24, 32-38, 40, 42, 45, 46, 48-50, 53, 55-60, 62-64, 66-68, 74, 124, 125, 128, 159, 164, 165, 167, 168, 170, 175, 178, 179, 201, 209
Infusion set 172
ISO 2, 3, 5-40, 42, 44-51, 53-57, 66, 67, 106-108, 115, 136, 137, 147, 164, 170, 186, 188, 192
ISO 10933 2
ISO 10993 106, 115, 117, 127, 132, 141, 142, 145, 147, 149, 152, 154-156, 158, 160, 162-165, 167-169

M

Macromolecules 1, 61
Margin of safety 116, 119, 124, 125, 158
Mechanical heart valve 10, 55, 63, 178, 201, 202, 209, 211, 217, 223
Medical devices 1, 2, 3, 5, 6, 20, 46, 53, 57, 69, 74, 105-108, 115, 117-119, 123-125, 127-130, 132, 146, 147, 149-155, 158-160, 163-165, 167-173, 192, 201, 202, 207, 217, 220
Metals 9, 32, 35, 46, 48, 63, 70, 107, 150, 168, 169, 202
Microscopy 68, 162, 163, 169, 173, 178, 203, 204, 206, 207, 209
Modeling 3, 113, 115, 125, 178, 179

O

Organotin 124

P

Pannus 175, 212, 216, 217, 221
Performance standards 74, 170, 171, 173
Phosphorylcholine 124, 125
Plastics 6, 8, 57-59, 66, 118, 180, 192
PMA 14, 15, 22, 27, 33, 42, 50, 54, 105, 127-131, 182, 183, 195
Polymers 1, 28, 30, 32, 45, 51, 53, 55, 57, 59, 66, 67, 70, 106, 107, 117-119, 124, 151, 152, 168, 169, 186, 194, 201, 202, 204
Polyurethane 6, 13, 14, 16, 19-21, 27, 28, 51, 55, 57, 71, 118, 123, 169
Preclinical testing 69, 74, 127, 128, 142
Product development 54, 118, 125, 127, 150, 181, 182, 184, 185, 187-190, 192, 193, 197, 198, 200
Proof testing 179
Properties 1-4, 6, 14, 30, 40, 42, 45, 46, 55, 56, 58-68, 107, 108, 120, 149, 166, 169, 178, 179, 190, 191, 201, 202, 206
Prototype 131, 172
Pyrogenicity 106, 114, 148, 149, 155, 159, 173

Q

Quality system 127-130, 145

R

Record keeping 181, 182, 184
Reproductive toxicity 5, 113, 147, 149, 160, 167, 168
Research 13, 14, 53, 105, 128, 130, 143-145, 194-196, 198, 200, 201, 208
RGD 202, 209, 217
Risk assessment 74, 107, 108, 113-115, 118, 119, 124, 125

S

Sensitization 5, 6, 107, 125, 141, 142, 153, 154, 173
Standards 2, 3, 5-51, 53-67, 74, 106-108, 125, 132, 144, 145, 147, 151, 155, 158, 170, 184, 188, 191, 195, 200
Sterilization 3-5, 51, 53, 55, 57-60, 63, 68, 107, 108, 111, 150, 170, 172, 182, 184, 189, 190, 193, 197, 202, 203, 207, 211, 212, 217, 220
Surface analysis 211
Surface modification 201, 202, 204, 206, 208
Systemic effect 6, 106, 112, 114, 125, 132, 141, 142, 148, 149, 155, 156, 158, 167, 173

T

Thrombus 4, 11, 24, 163, 166, 178, 202, 209, 212, 216
Tissue 1-4, 11, 13, 20-22, 24, 25, 27, 28, 30, 32, 33, 40, 42, 46, 47, 53, 55, 57-60, 63, 70, 73, 106, 107, 113, 116, 118, 120, 121, 123, 125, 132, 137, 148, 149, 152, 153, 155, 159, 163-165, 167-170, 175, 178, 194-202, 206-208, 212, 217
Tissue engineering 194, 195, 198, 200
Toxicity 3, 5, 6, 20, 106, 107, 111-116, 119-121, 124, 125, 141, 142, 147-149, 151, 153, 155, 158, 160, 165, 167, 168, 170, 173, 199, 200, 206
Toxicokinetic 6, 116, 119, 149, 169, 170, 173
Tripartite 2, 132

V

Validation 54, 55, 131, 145, 151, 172, 181, 183-185, 187, 189, 190
Vascular graft 13, 19, 61, 63, 107, 108, 118, 124, 150, 166, 167, 170, 174, 178, 179, 198, 207-209
Vascular patch 203, 208, 217, 218, 220
Vendor relationships 182
Vertical standards 107

X

XPS 203, 204, 211, 212, 217

[redacted]